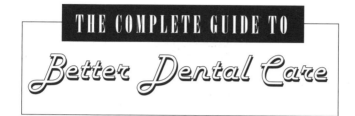

THE COMPLETE GUIDE TO
Better Dental Care

THE COMPLETE GUIDE TO

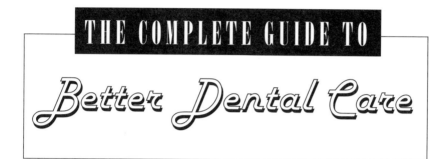

Better Dental Care

Jerry F. Taintor, D.D.S., M.S.
Mary Jane Taintor

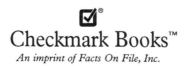

Checkmark Books™
An imprint of Facts On File, Inc.

The Complete Guide to Better Dental Care

First paperback printing 1999

Copyright © 1997 by Jerry F. Taintor and Mary Jane Taintor

Checkmark Books
An imprint of Facts On File, Inc.
11 Penn Plaza
New York NY 10001

Library of Congress Cataloging-in-Publication Data

Taintor, Jerry F.
The complete guide to better dental care /
Jerry F. Taintor, Mary Jane Taintor
p. cm.
Includes index.
ISBN 0-8160-3383-8 (hc)
ISBN 0-8160-4005-2 (pb)
1. Dentistry—Popular works. 2. Consumer education. I. Taintor.
Mary Jane. II. Title.
RK61.T147 1997
617.6—dc21   96-51103

You can find Facts On File on the World Wide Web at
http://www.factsonfile.com

Text and cover design by Cathy Rincon
Layout by Robert Yaffe
Cover photograph by Arnold Katz
Illustrations on pages 69, 184, and 219 by Jeremy Eagle

Printed in the United States of America

MP FOF 10 9 8 7 6 5 4 3 2
(pbk) 10 9 8 7 6 5 4 3 2 1

This book is printed on acid-free paper.

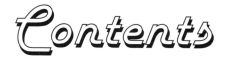

Contents

PART II: THE DENTAL SPECIALTIES   61

PART III: TRENDS, FEARS, AND ISSUES IN DENTISTRY   151

To our daughter, Christy

Preface

The purpose of this book is to help foster communication between dental professionals and their patients. Hopefully, this communication will lead to better dental care for you, the patient. A good dental consumer knows the questions to ask and has a general knowledge of what to look for in the care he is receiving from his dentist. Do you think the amateur car buffs get better service from their mechanic since they know what is happening and can talk over the problem with the mechanic in the mechanic's own terms? Sure they do! But there are very few "amateur dental buffs." These amateurs are almost exclusively limited to dental assistants, dental receptionists, or dental hygienists. Now people outside of the dental profession have the opportunity to play an active role in improving the quality of their own dental health care.

At the time of this writing, dental products alone represent approximately a $2 billion national expense, and dental services represent another public expenditure above $38.5 billion. That is a great deal of money, with many different enterprising companies trying to get a piece of the action. Studies have shown that the average person spends between 30 seconds and one minute a day maintaining his or her dental health (brushing, flossing, etc.). Outside of exposure to toothbrush and toothpaste advertisements very little time is spent thinking about teeth. At the same time most people use their teeth at least three times a day for meals; to communicate, to improve their appearance, to help secure a job or mate; and even to breathe through these same teeth; and they wonder, for social reasons, if their breath odor is in some way related to the condition of their teeth. Most people would agree that teeth are very important; however, most will agree that they know next to nothing about teeth other than that they should be brushed at least once a day. For most people the primary focus of attention on teeth is when they hurt because this interferes with their normal daily life.

What makes the situation seem out of control for most individuals is that, outside of this book, little public information of any substance is readily available to help a consumer make a logical or informed decision about spending hard-earned money for dental care or dental products.

This book can be used either as a programmed textbook or as a reference book. As a programmed text, the book will help you develop a working vocabulary of dental terminology and concepts as you read the chapters in consecutive order. Technical words are highlighted. A glossary of terms in the back of the book will help refresh your memory if you cannot remember the meaning of a technical word. For those who want to use the book as a reference text, a reference index is provided that lists pages in the book where a particular term is used and explained in different contexts. The latest fee information available for different areas of the United States and Canada has also been included in this book.

This book deals with the issues of spending money for dental care and products, and knowing your money is being spent wisely. It also helps you, the consumer, understand the nature of services rendered for your benefit. Many times consumers with limited information rely on friends and family whose base of information is limited to their own personal experiences. With the advent of all the managed-care dental insurance in this country it is even more important for dental patients to be good dental consumers. When it is time for you to choose your dental plan at work you need to understand what benefits best suit the needs of you and your family. Very significant changes have taken place in dentistry since the first edition of this book, and new technology will continue to affect dentistry in the future.

This is the book to read if you want to maintain your teeth and minimize your costs through proper home care and appropriate services provided to you. This includes everyone from those who have their teeth and what to keep them; those with only some of their teeth remaining who want to keep what they have and possibly replace what is missing; and those who have no natural teeth. This means you!

Acknowledgments

We would like to give special thanks to everyone who has offered both their support and valued opinions. Throughout the course of researching for this book many people have been contacted for information. Without their input this book would not have been possible. Special thanks goes to Dr. and Mrs. George Hansen, Drs. Tom and Jerri Munn, Dr. Bob Biesterfeld, Dr. Leonard Andre, Dr. Ahmad Fahid, and Dr. Andy Slisco for all their time and effort to make sure the book is complete and accurate.

PART I

The Consumer and the General Dentist

1

Dental Fitness = Prevention

itness implies prevention. Health is determined by biological, behavioral, social, economic, and environmental factors. Today there is an emphasis on individuals actively assuming a larger share of responsibility for their own good health and depending less on the health-care professional. In order to prevent health problems we must change our smoking, eating, exercise, and oral health habits.

Americans are now realizing that sound oral health is an essential part of total health and physical well-being. As a result of preventive dental programs and an increased awareness of good dental health, tooth decay in schoolchildren dropped 32 percent in the decade of the 1970s, and the proportion of children completely free of dental decay has risen almost 10 percent since 1973. Adults have also benefited. The latest statistics show that only 40 percent of the adult population is in need of either full or partial dentures.

Since the 1950s, the focus in the dental profession has been on prevention. Regular visits and long-term patient care by the dentist have resulted in successful preventive care. Teeth with little or no decay are not necessarily an indication that your mouth is in a healthy condition. This point cannot be emphasized enough. At regular checkups dentists look for gum disease, decay, tumors, abscesses on the root tips of the teeth (as seen only by X rays), and the general health of the mouth. The dentist uses his professional experience and X rays to diagnose these problems. Regular checkups allow small problems to be corrected before they become serious. Poor dental health not only affects the way you feel and look, but it also leads to serious health complications such as infections in your body and even oral cancer.

In between regular, routine visits to the dentist, each of us must take personal responsibility to promote oral health. We must see our dentist regularly, brush and floss daily, eat a balanced diet that is low in refined sugar, limit snacks between meals, and use toothpaste and mouthwash that contain fluoride. If you live in an area that has the correct amount of fluoride in the water system (one part fluoride per 1 million parts water) you will receive extra protection against tooth decay. Studies have indicated that the most dramatic decrease in the incidence of tooth decay in the United States is a result of fluoridated municipal water systems.

Healthy teeth not only enable you to look good, feel good, and have a good mental attitude about yourself, but they also make it possible to eat and speak properly without discomfort. Good oral health is important to your total health.

Like all things in nature, our teeth and their supportive structures tend to break down in time. Not all teeth or supportive structures deteriorate at an equal rate, and consumers need information on two levels: what they can do for themselves, and what dentists can and should do for their patients, both before and after problems arise.

Most conflicts and confusions occur when the patient's expectations are not in harmony with the dentist's expectations. The more information available to the consumer, however, the greater the chance that consumers and their dentists will communicate effectively.

To achieve good oral health, you may need to see a general dentist or a dental specialist, depending on the problem. To make an intelligent decision, you need to know the scope of expertise of both the general dentist and the specialist. What each has to offer is the subject of the following chapters.

HOW TO CHOOSE A DENTIST

One problem that practically everyone faces is how to go about finding a "good" dentist. Most people make this crucial decision several times during their lives. As a consumer, there are several aspects you should consider about your dentist and his office after you have decided on a particular dentist to care for your teeth.

The phone book is filled with dentists who all have one thing in common: a license to practice dentistry in your state. However, they all have different personalities, different levels of experience, and different degrees of expertise. Before you begin looking for a dentist, you should ask yourself these questions:

1. Are you looking for a dentist near your home, or are you willing to travel a reasonable distance to be treated by a particular dentist you trust and like?
2. Are certain times of the day or week better for you? Some dentists have early or late office hours; some work on Saturdays. How important are these considerations?
3. Do you have a physical handicap that requires special attention? Some general dentists and certain specialists cater to specific problems. Also, handicapped patients may need to consider the physical layout of the dental office and its location in relation to parking.
4. What is your problem? Do you need your teeth cleaned and checked? Do you have an emergency? These factors will determine whether you need to see someone immediately or whether you can wait for a regular scheduled appointment.
5. Do you need a general dentist or a specialist? General dentists are trained to do all types of treatment; however, if you have difficult or unusual problems, the general dentist may refer you to a specialist.

The most readily available sources of information about dentists are your friends, acquaintances, work associates, family physician, or pharmacist. Ask them how long they have gone to their dentist, and how they made their selection. You will primarily find out something about these dentists' personalities, but you should realize that you will rarely get much information about their technical abilities.

Another way to find a dentist is to call your local dental society (see appendix C for state dental societies). It can be located by looking in the Yellow Pages under "dentist." They can assist you by recommending several dentists in your area who seem to fit your needs. Then you can call these dentists and decide for yourself if you feel comfortable. You may also want to check on the credentials of a particular dentist. For example, you may want to know if the dentist providing orthodontic treatment is a specialist or a general dentist. Your local dental society can also help you find a dentist if you have an emergency situation. Most societies have rotating emergency lists of dentists who have volunteered to take dental emergency calls on a 24-hour basis.

If you are moving, your current dentist is an excellent person to ask for a recommendation. Many times, if he does not know anyone, he will have a colleague who can give him a recommendation.

Several aspects of the dentist's practice can give you useful information in making your choice.

1. Is the dentist and/or his hygienist prevention oriented, pointing out things you can do yourself in order to maintain good dental health? The dentist and/or his hygienist should provide *oral prophylaxis*

(tooth cleaning), fluoride treatments, sealants, replacements for missing teeth, and needed *restorations* (fillings). Home care is up to you.

2. Does he or she emphasize continued long-term care? In other words, is there a recall system that automatically notifies you when it's time for your periodic checkup?

3. Does the dentist use dental X rays, when needed, to assist in diagnosing your problem? On the initial visits to his office, he should request that you have X rays taken of all your teeth so he can determine the overall condition of your mouth. On subsequent visits X rays should be taken as needed. No dentist should restore a tooth without proper X rays. At the time of the X ray, note if the dentist is radiation conscious. He should place a lead apron over you to protect you from any "scatter radiation." He should even have a thyroid collar on the lead-lined apron.

Using the information from the X rays and other diagnostic parameters of evaluation, a dentist can suggest what treatment is needed to restore your mouth to good condition again. This is a far better and less expensive route for you to take than just "taking care of what hurts." Dental problems are much less expensive to treat in their early stages. More about X rays will be discussed later.

4. Does the dentist take a complete medical and dental history to be included as part of your permanent record? This gives the dentist insight into your particular needs. It can also help prevent possible complications. For instance, it would alert the dentist to allergies you might have to medicines, or to an illness that might require modification of the usual treatment. Even if you have gone to this particular dentist regularly for a period of time, you should be sure that he is aware of any changes in your medical status, medicines you might be using now, or allergies that might have been detected since your last visit. Do not make the decision on your own that any medical information is of no dental significance. Let your dentist make this decision. For example, you might recently have found that you are a diabetic. This is significant to your dentist, even though the disease has no apparent direct involvement with your teeth. The reason is that diabetes causes a delay in the healing process. Diabetes also can cause *gingivitis* (gum inflammation). This may mean you need to make more frequent visits to his office to have your teeth cleaned.

5. Does the dentist or his staff openly discuss your treatment needs, fees, and payment plans in advance of treatment? This approach allows both parties' expectations to be met, and fosters a lasting relationship.

6. Is emergency care available? Though many dentists list their home telephone numbers, others have answering services. Usually, an answering service takes calls and helps you find either your own dentist or someone who has agreed to handle after-hours emergency calls. Some dental societies have a list of volunteer dentists who will meet your emergency needs on a 24-hour basis.

The most important step in finding a dentist, however, is to look *before* you need one, not after you have no choice but to take whoever is available.

CHEAP DENTISTRY VS. INEXPENSIVE DENTISTRY

"How much do you charge for a filling in a back tooth?" the caller asks the receptionist. She explains that it depends on what is wrong and what treatment is needed. Looking at the tooth as a box with five sides (tooth surfaces), it depends on how many of the surfaces need to be restored. The more surfaces in need of repair, the more extensive, and hence, the more expensive the treatment. You might only need a single chewing surface restoration (filling). The cost for this treatment will be relatively nominal.

The other extreme is that the tooth may be so badly decayed that there are no surfaces left to the box except the bottom, as when the tooth is decayed down to the gum line. Usually, no restoration, by itself, will take care of this situation. This tooth will need root canal therapy, posts cemented into one or more of the root canals, rebuilding the tooth using the posts for length, and, finally, a cap (technically termed a *crown*) placed over the buildup to restore the tooth to its original form and function. In addition, surgical intervention may be necessary to remove extensive infection at the end of the root. This treatment could cost well over a thousand dollars in many areas of the country.

Shopping by telephone for the least expensive dental fees will not get you the answer you are really seeking. In the long run, the cheapest services could eventually be much more expensive. As I have already pointed out, the best approach is to establish a relationship with a dentist and see him on a regular basis for preventive care. This will make it unnecessary for most expensive dental treatment because problems are caught early.

But if you don't have a dentist, the next best thing is to choose one and make an appointment for a consultation. It is always a good idea to get an estimate *before* you begin, but realize that money is not the most important aspect of your dental treatment. In today's competitive market, the cost of services really do not vary that much in a specific area, but the quality of care you receive can vary. Getting an estimate is your way of screening the dentist. A dentist must do two things to give you an estimate: not only do a visual exam of your mouth and teeth, but also take a series of X rays of your teeth and bone to disclose problems you might have that are hidden from eyesight. For example, X rays show decay between teeth or reveal abscessed (infected) teeth that might not even be painful at this time.

When you get an estimate from your dentist, ask for a written, itemized treatment plan along with the costs. If you feel that this is the dentist for you and that his treatment alternatives are within your budget, then do not wait to proceed with treatment. Get your teeth restored before they get worse! I have yet to see dental treatment get less extensive with time.

If you decide to seek a second opinion, which no dentist should object to, the best protocol is to ask the first dentist to send your X rays to the office of the second dentist. Presuming the first dentist took X rays of adequate quality and quantity, the second dentist should be able to use them, thus eliminating extra cost and needless radiation exposure to you. You should then need only a visual exam for the second dentist to provide you with a written, itemized treatment plan along with costs. Again, you must go to the dentist's office before he can give you an estimate. Compare the two estimates. If both dentists are located in the same area of your city, the fee for the same services should be similar.

It is important to recognize the difference between "cheap" and "inexpensive" dentistry. In my opinion, cheap dental estimates are those that leave out major necessary treatment to make the cost estimate low. Inexpensive dentistry is dentistry that not only is comparable with the average charges for these services in your area but also includes all the treatment you need to eliminate your problems.

In choosing a treatment plan for yourself, it is important to look at the long-term needs of your teeth. Many people tend to want to take care of only what hurts and let the rest go until they experience pain again. In the long run, this is detrimental to your health and teeth, and it results in even more costly dental treatment.

As a consumer, you should read and compare your treatment plans carefully. Focus on the major items such as periodontal therapy (gum disease treatment), root canal therapy, gold and porcelain crowns, etc. For example, if one estimate says you need periodontal therapy and the other doesn't, you may want to get still another opinion from a specialist in the particular area in question. For your reference, I have included what you might expect to pay for dental treatment in your area in the Dental Fees chapter.

Be aware that many times insurance companies let the *cost* of services, not what services are best for you, dictate what they will authorize for payment. This is particularly true of the managed-care plans. Don't be fooled into thinking that just because the insurance company will not pay for a particular service then it must not be the best thing for you to have in your mouth. Remember that insurance companies are as profit motivated as any other business.

In the end, the decision is a personal one. It is your decision about who will treat you. If you want a healthy mouth, it is very important to get a correct diagnosis of what your dental problems are and then have them treated. It could mean the difference between keeping or losing your tooth (or teeth)!

TEETH: FORM AND FUNCTION

In reply to your innocent question "What's wrong with my tooth?" your dentist may open up a rapid-fire explanation along these lines: "The X rays of your teeth indicate that your lower left second molar has a decayed area on the mesial. Right now the decay extends through the enamel and is into the dentin. If you do not get it restored soon, the caries will eventually invade the pulp. Then your tooth will require root canal therapy. In addition, the gums have receded in that same area. Your brushing has removed some of the cementum and exposed the dentin. That is why your teeth are sensitive."

Your immediate response would probably be: "Oh! So what should I do?" But do you really know what the dentist said? You might know which tooth since it is sensitive every time that you have a cold or hot drink. But his explanation of your dental problem may sound like a foreign language. What is enamel, dentin, cementum . . . and where is the pulp?

His foreign language is technical dental terminology. The words may be only vaguely familiar to you, depending on your familiarity with dentistry. At this point in the discussion with your dentist, you may not really be sure if you should be worried or relieved.

You may at one time have had to memorize the parts of a tooth for a biology class, but that did not have any real significance for you at the time. So now for a refresher course! Let us take a look at the basic components of a tooth so that you can talk about, and even understand, the information your dentist may be trying to tell you.

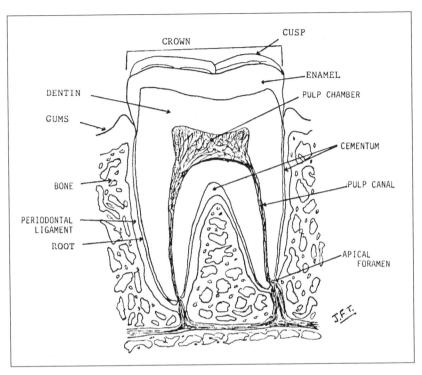

Figure 1

The drawing [figure 1] is that of a lower molar. That is one of the teeth farthest back in the lower jaw.

Essentially, all your teeth are composed of the same basic parts. First let us examine the structure of the tooth closely, and then let us relate this to their function. As with modern architecture, the basic premise is "form follows function."

The tooth structure protruding out of the gum tissue is the crown. This part of the tooth is divided into surfaces. The easiest way to understand this concept is to compare the crown of the tooth to a box, which has four sides and a top. The surface of the tooth closest to the midline is the *mesial*. The surface opposite of the midline is the *distal*. The surface on the tongue side of the tooth is the *lingual*. The surface on the cheek side of the tooth is the *buccal*. The top (chewing surface) of the tooth is called the *occlusal*.

The crown of every tooth is totally covered with *enamel*. Enamel is the hardest, most mineralized tissue in the body, and without it, the inner part of the tooth would be quickly worn away by chewing. It is in this outermost layer of the tooth that decay penetrates to make its way inside the tooth.

Under the enamel is another layer of the tooth called the *dentin*. If dental decay is able to gnaw its way though the enamel, it next attacks the dentin. Softer than enamel, dentin is more like bone. It is composed of millions of tiny tubules that lead directly to the dental pulp (see below). Dentin forms the bulk of the entire tooth from the crown to the *root*.

The root is almost entirely composed of dentin, with the exception of another thin layer of bonelike tissue covering the outer root surface below the gum line in healthy teeth. This thin layer is the *cementum*.

The supportive tissues of the tooth are collectively called the *periodontium*. It includes the periodontal ligament, *gingiva* (gums), and bone that supports the tooth. If you think of the tooth as a house, the periodontium is the foundation of that house.

Between the jawbone and the cementum is the *periodontal ligament (PDL)*. The PDL is a strong fiberlike tissue that connects the root's cementum (and hence the root) to the jawbone.

Proper care of the gingiva is important because they can become inflamed by bacteria and other irritants. The inflammation, if it continues, can cause gums to recede (pull away from teeth) and allow bacteria to spread to the bone. The bone then *resorbs* (is dissolved away). This results in the destruction of the bone supporting the teeth. When this occurs, the teeth become loose and may eventually fall out or need to be removed. This, not dental decay, is the number one cause of teeth being lost today. This disease is called *periodontitis*. If the foundation (or periodontium) is weak, the result can be the loss of the best constructed house (or tooth).

Dental decay, if left to destroy the enamel and dentin, will eventually infect or even kill the pulp tissue in the center of the tooth.

The *pulp* is a soft tissue found in the center of all teeth. It is composed of blood vessels, fibers, cells, and nerve tissue. *Caries* (decay) usually first extends into the *pulp chamber* (the space inside the crown of the tooth where the pulp is located). At this point, you usually feel pain. Generally, the pain may be accompanied by swelling from infection, which is referred to as an *abscess*. The pain may be spontaneous or occur as the result of taking in hot, cold, or sweet foods or fluids. It usually lingers for some period of time.

The pulp chamber is located in the lowermost portion of the tooth's crown and extends down each root. The space the pulp occupies in the root is called the pulp canal or, more commonly, the *root canal*.

The root canal ends at the *apex* (end) of the root of the tooth at the *apical foramen*. This is where the pulp tissue exits the tooth into the jawbone and becomes neuro-vascular tissue (nerve and blood vessels). When the pulp is diseased, it has to be removed in order to save the tooth. The space is then cleaned, shaped, filed, and filled. This is called *root canal therapy.* The whole area of endodontics will be discussed in chapter 3.

Now let us examine the function of your teeth [figures 2 and 3]. The part of the tooth you see when you look in your bathroom mirror is the *crown.* The crown determines the tooth's function. The crowns of the front teeth, the *incisors* (the four front teeth, upper and lower), are sharp and chisel-shaped for cutting (or incising). The next tooth back in the

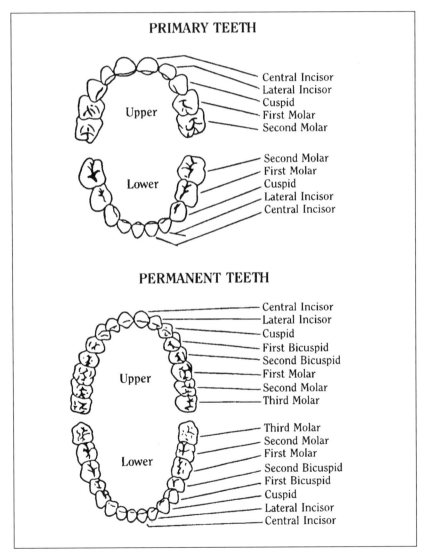

PRIMARY TEETH

Upper
- Central Incisor
- Lateral Incisor
- Cuspid
- First Molar
- Second Molar

Lower
- Second Molar
- First Molar
- Cuspid
- Lateral Incisor
- Central Incisor

PERMANENT TEETH

Upper
- Central Incisor
- Lateral Incisor
- Cuspid
- First Bicuspid
- Second Bicuspid
- First Molar
- Second Molar
- Third Molar

Lower
- Third Molar
- Second Molar
- First Molar
- Second Bicuspid
- First Bicuspid
- Cuspid
- Lateral Incisor
- Central Incisor

Figure 2

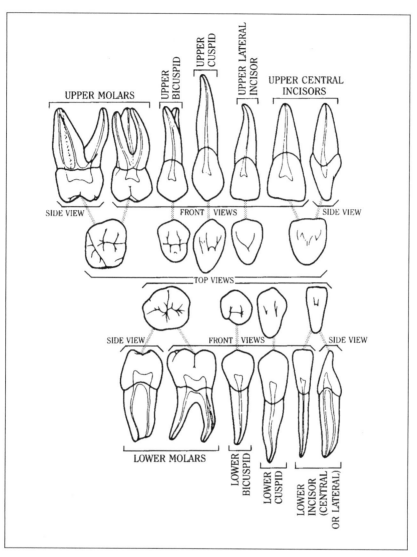

Figure 3

mouth is the *cuspid* (or *canine tooth*). These have pointed *cusps* on the biting surface for tearing. The *premolars*, the next two teeth back in the mouth, usually have two cusps on their biting surface; hence, they are sometimes referred to as bicuspids. The premolars are for crushing and tearing. Finally, the farthest two teeth back (three teeth back if you have your wisdom teeth) are the *molars*. These have several cusps on the biting surface and are used for grinding. All together there are 32 permanent (adult) teeth. Children have 20 deciduous (baby) teeth.

You have just had a crash course in the basic parts, types, and functions of the teeth.

Now go back to the beginning of this section and see for yourself if the conversation between the hypothetical patient and the dentist makes more sense.

ADA SEAL OF ACCEPTANCE

Companies competing for their share of the $2 billion market in dental products go to great lengths to bring their products to the dental professionals' and consumers' attention. Partly in the interest of goodwill and partly out of self-interest, these companies spend millions of dollars on dental research, educational projects, grants, and fellowships, as well as many other ventures that would not otherwise be accomplished. This has resulted in improved dental products.

The American Dental Association (ADA) is the largest and most widely recognized organization in the United States for dentists. Its purpose is to serve as a governing body for its members and to promote quality dental care. The ADA Council on Scientific Affairs grants the *ADA Seal* [see figure 4] when a product meets all the ADA's requirements for safety and efficacy. Consumers and dentists have relied on the stringent guidelines and standards required of recipients of the ADA Seal for selecting safe, effective dental products since 1930. The ADA Seal is the *only* labeling on dental products that assures the consumer of safety and efficacy and that the manufacturer's claims are true. Only products that have been granted the Seal may display it on their products. Participation in the Seal program is voluntary.

It is very important to understand the difference between the ADA Seal and the Federal Drug Administration (FDA) license to market drugs and dental materials/devices. In therapeutics, FDA approval of a drug does not necessarily address dental applications of the previously FDA-approved drug, and not every therapeutic agent must be submitted for FDA scrutiny. Regarding materials and devices, the FDA encourages organizations such as the ADA to offer voluntary standards because its own mandatory standards program is relatively new and far less comprehensive when it comes to dental materials and devices. *It is very important to understand that the FDA does not address the safety and efficacy of dental*

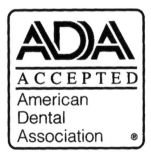

Figure 4

materials and devices. They only give permission to market these types of products. The ADA Seal is the best assurance consumers and professionals have that drugs, materials, and devices have met guidelines for safety and efficacy, and that the claims being made by the manufacturer are indeed true.

The ADA Seal program is respected throughout the world, and looked at as a model. Dr. Ken Burrell, Senior Director, ADA Council on Scientific Affairs, states "Practitioners in other countries invariably remark on the fact they prefer to buy a product with the ADA Seal, even though it sometimes can be difficult and expensive for them to order these items."

Over 300 over-the-counter products (toothpastes, mouthwashes, toothbrushes, etc.) and 850 professional and prescription products carry the Seal. All products go through the same basic process before receiving the Seal. They must first demonstrate safety and effectiveness by meeting specific ADA guidelines and standards. And, of course, all submissions must include results from clinical studies proving the product does what it claims to do—such as fighting decay, reducing gingivitis, or decreasing sensitivity in teeth. Submissions are often sent to outside consultants for review. Over 150 experts in all areas of dentistry serve as volunteer consultants. The ADA ensures impartiality of its consultants by requiring them to disclose any potential conflicts of interest.

The process can take weeks, or even months. The laboratory staff of the Council on Scientific Affairs tests about 100 new products each year. In addition, the laboratories test about 100 products each year that are under consideration for continued acceptance. Manufacturers must reapply for the Seal for their products every three years. And if ADA standards or guidelines change, the manufacturer must submit data showing the product complies with the new requirements, sometimes immediately and sometimes upon the three-year renewal.

Wayne Wozniak, Ph.D, Director of Evaluation Criteria at the ADA Council on Scientific Affairs, states "We review our standards every five years. If materials for a product have improved, for example, the standards may become more stringent to keep pace with the state of the art of that product." Dr. Wozniak states that about 30 percent of products initially fail the materials laboratory tests.

Finally, after a product has met all the guidelines, it is brought before the Council on Scientific Affairs, which meets three times a year. About 20 submissions are considered at each meeting, and approximately 90 percent of the products submitted for consideration are eventually given the Seal (but not until they meet all the criteria for safety and effectiveness). Sometimes a manufacturer must submit a product several times, after making improvements or redesigning it, before it is granted the ADA Seal.

After the Council gives the ADA Seal, the Council's Advertising Review Committee checks all the product's advertising, labeling, and packaging. The ADA's goal is to ensure that all promotional claims are scientifically sound. This is balanced against the manufacturer's need to market the product creatively.

Dr. Burrell states "the Acceptance Program helps ensure that dental products for professional and over-the-counter use are what they are claimed to be." Dentists who use products with the ADA Seal can be assured the product is high quality. Patients can trust that these products will meet their claims.

The least expensive and simplest approach to the problem of making sure you have bought wisely when you purchase a dental product is to look for the ADA Seal. *Always buy products with the ADA Seal to insure that the product has been tested for safety and efficacy, and that the manufacturer's claims are true.*

HOME CARE

For most of the 20th century the major emphasis in dentistry has been on the avoidance of dental caries. Now dental professionals are realizing they need to focus on preventive maintenance of periodontal disease. The techniques exist to eliminate virtually all local factors (plaque and calculus) responsible for periodontal disease.

Good oral health requires a team effort between yourself and your general dentist and his staff. In order for it to be successful you must realize that only *you* can make the effort a success. The outcome will depend on how well you clean your teeth and gingiva (gums) each day. A healthy diet is also important.

Home care involves the use of a toothbrush, toothpaste, mouthwash, floss, toothpicks, and possibly an oral irrigating device. Good home care is the backbone of preventing dental disease. Brushing and flossing are the two primary methods of providing good home care for you and your children. As the ADA Seal of Acceptance states, brushing with an approved toothpaste "can be of significant value when used in a conscientiously applied program of oral hygiene." The "program" is one you must orchestrate in conjunction with your dentist.

Your dentist provides you with regular dental checkups (taking X rays when necessary) to detect decay and periodontal disease. If there are any weak points in your home care, your dentist can intervene and correct the situation before it gets to a point of urgency. His intervention involves recognizing and treating problems that you are not trained to see. Either he or his hygienist provides a thorough cleaning of your teeth on a regular basis to prevent periodontal disease. Many times pit-and-fissure sealants are placed on children's teeth to help prevent decay. In conjunction with this care, the dentist or one of his staff members will provide you with instructions on how to do your home care. Once you begin active home care, the staff will serve as a resource for you if you have questions or problems.

In general, dental examinations are usually done every six to twelve months. Some patients, however, need to see the dentist more often. The dentist determines this based on your *DMF index*—a way of counting how many of your teeth are decayed (D), missing (M), or filled (F). It also depends on how quickly you build up *calculus* (tartar).

Studies show there are two myths that commonly lead to a lapse in home care. Patients who have been successful in reversing a periodontal problem with a preventive care program sometimes believe that some permanent immunity has been created. In addition, some patients who have completed periodontal therapy may feel they have been "cured" with no possibility for recurrence. Both of these beliefs are false.

When dental professionals focus on prevention it allows periodontal disease to be intercepted with relatively simple procedures. This reduces the need for complicated treatment options caused by delayed diagnosis.

Today, preventive dentistry is considered a standard of dental practice. It is the primary way to ensure that good dental health and quality care are maintained over a lifetime. If preventive education is minimized or omitted, most dental professionals would consider this substandard care.

A healthy mouth projects an attractive smile that is noticed by all. A person who takes care of his teeth and gums reflects a person who values himself.

Diet and Dental Health

In addition to daily brushing, flossing, and using a mouth rinse, it is important to eat a balanced diet so that your body can get the nutrients needed for good health. The U.S. Department of Agriculture advises eating six to eleven servings of breads and cereals, three to five servings of vegetables, two to four servings of fruit, two to three servings of dairy products, and two servings of meat, poultry, fish, eggs, beans, or nuts each day.

If your diet is low in the nutrients you need it will be hard for you to resist infection in the tissues of your mouth, which can contribute to *periodontal* (gum) disease. If children do not have a balanced diet their teeth may not develop properly. In order for them to develop strong, decay-resistant teeth, they need a balanced diet with emphasis on calcium, phosphorous, and proper levels of fluoride.

Your eating patterns and food choices are important factors in helping to reduce caries (decay) in your teeth. The reason is that everything you eat passes through your mouth. When you eat foods that contain carbohydrates (sugars and starches), the bacteria in plaque produce acids that can destroy tooth enamel. After repeated attacks, the tooth enamel begins to break down, forming a cavity.

In addition to white or brown refined sugar (*sucrose*), there are several other different kinds of sugars that are harmful to your teeth. These include *fructose* (fruit sugar), glucose, lactose (milk sugar), and *maltose* (grain sugar). Foods that contain sucrose naturally are beets, melons, bananas, sweet potatoes, and peaches. Other foods that contain one or more of the above sugars are apples, raisins, milk, grapes, and pears. Even the syrup from some liquid medications contains sugars. Processed foods that have sugar added are catsup, peanut butter, and salad dressing. People who use "natural" sweeteners such as honey, molasses, or corn sweeteners should realize that these sweeteners all can contribute to tooth decay.

In recent years dental researchers have learned that foods that contain starches can also cause the bacteria in plaque to produce acid. Foods that contain starches include breads, cereals, processed foods, fruits, and vegetables. Many researchers believe that if starchy foods (especially those that also contain sugar) are left on the teeth or in the mouth for any length of time they can be dentally harmful.

It is important to remember that the acids in foods that contain carbohydrates attack your teeth for 20 minutes or more after you eat. The more often you eat these foods, the more acid attacks you have. Therefore, you should limit the number of times you eat snacks between meals. Try *not* to eat foods such as hard candies, breath mints, or cough drops, all of which stay in the mouth for extended periods of time. Foods that contain carbohydrates are less harmful if eaten with a meal because the saliva production is increased during this time. Saliva helps rinse food from the mouth. Some researchers feel that certain foods such as cheese, peanuts, or sugar-free chewing gum help counter the effects of the acids produced by the bacteria in plaque when carbohydrates are eaten.

All patients who have eating disorders (even those who do not binge-eat or vomit) are at increased risk for abnormal dental erosion. Several patients in a recent study reported that they avoided dental treatment out of fear that the dentist would detect an eating disorder when he saw the erosion of the enamel in the teeth.

Good dental health depends on more than diet alone. You must brush, floss, and use fluoride daily. These measures can reduce dental disease. Be sure to also visit your dentist regularly.

Toothbrushes

To be successful, good oral hygiene has to be practiced on an ongoing basis at home. Prevention begins at your own bathroom, where you brush and floss thoroughly each day. Brushing not only removes plaque, but also massages the gingiva (gums). The effectiveness of any preventive program is measured by the patient's level of compliance and their ability to manipulate the toothbrush, floss, etc., correctly.

You probably have been told to brush after every meal, and whenever possible, after every snack. This is still ideal. You should comply with this suggestion, particularly if your teeth are prone to decay or if you have periodontal disease. In some cases, however, differing recommendations are warranted. Factors to consider include the patient's diet, overall oral health and susceptibility to oral disease, and the presence of physical conditions such as decreased saliva flow. Most studies indicate that early-morning brushing is universally indicated because the body's natural plaque fighters are less active during sleep, so plaque accumulates more quickly. For the same reason it is advisable to brush and floss before retiring to reduce the number of bacteria in and around the teeth during this time of lessened natural defense.

Buying a toothbrush can be as confusing as deciding on a pair of new shoes. The variety of shapes and sizes staggers the imagination. Brushes are divided into two categories—manual and powered. Manual brushes come in every color and size, and have bristles that are rippled, trimmed to a dome shape, and available in several neon colors. You can get brushes with handles that have a non-slip grip and a flexible neck that enables it to bend as you brush. There are even brushes on the market with handles that are activated by the heat from the user's hand to change colors.

The best toothbrush is one that the patient will use. Dr. Wayne Wozniak, director of the ADA Council on Scientific Affairs, states that "as long as a toothbrush has soft, end-rounded bristles and removes plaque, the ADA takes no position on whether certain bristles or handles are better than others." The size and choice of style of a brush is determined not only by the size of the patient's mouth but also by the patient's age and manual dexterity.

Sonic and ultrasonic toothbrushes, which have been recently introduced on the market, are classified as manual brushes. They emit waves to vibrate the bristles at high frequencies. This makes these brushes very effective for removing plaque and stains. Standard manual brushing techniques can be employed with these brushes, which utilize rechargable batteries. The Sonicare toothbrush is available with a two-minute timer. This is a particularly nice feature for those who have a tendency to rush, because it encourages you to continue brushing until the timer stops.

Power toothbrushes usually have a small brush head. Even though this limits the number of teeth the brush covers at any one time in an area, the design allows the user increased access to less accessible areas. No one has ever proven that electric toothbrushes clean teeth better than conventional brushes when properly used. An electric toothbrush may, however, be the best choice if you have dexterity problems or a physical disability.

Before you consider purchasing a brush be sure it has the ADA Seal. This is the only way to be sure that it has been tested for safety and efficacy, and that the claims made by the manufacturer are true.

A dry brush does a more thorough job of cleaning than a wet brush. Thus, the ADA suggests that you have two toothbrushes. That way, you can always have one drying.

A toothbrush should be replaced after no more than three to four months of use. Look for frayed or bent bristles that are broken or worn. These are sure signs that a toothbrush should be replaced. In addition, when you see toothpaste clogged around the bristles' base, this is another sign that the toothbrush must be replaced. A worn-out toothbrush does not effectively clean off dental plaque that leads to tooth decay and periodontal problems. The bent and broken bristles can injure your gingiva. The small cost of a replacement is too insignificant to warrant the risk of damage from a worn-out toothbrush.

Proper brushing usually takes about three to four minutes. It depends on the clinical conditions in the mouth and the patient's dexterity in using the brush. Most people reach an ideal time spent on brushing through trial and error. You can check how well you have done by using a *disclosing solution*. This is a dye that stains any areas where plaque has been left after brushing. Disclosing solutions can be found in the "dental needs" section of most drugstores. The time you spend brushing can be increased if there seem to be areas you are missing.

There are several accepted methods for brushing teeth. You need to consult your dentist to determine which method is best for you. One very effective method is as follows: To brush the outer surfaces of the teeth, place the brush at a 45-degree angle to the gums. Then gently move the brush back and forth in short strokes no longer than half a tooth. A soft bristle brush will clean under the gums without injuring them. Still using the short scrubbing motion, concentrate on the inside surfaces of the teeth. This is where most neglect has been shown to occur. Use the "toe" of the brush to clean the inner front tooth surfaces. Complete your brushing by using short back-and-forth strokes on the chewing surfaces of the teeth. Make sure you do not miss any teeth or tooth surfaces.

One hint: Brush your tongue. Really! Brushing the tongue cleans off oral microorganisms that contribute to bad breath. Some periodontists even suggest that you brush the inside of your cheeks. Do this gently, of course. The whole idea is to minimize or eliminate as many oral bacteria as possible.

Regardless of the method you use, a systematic sequence of brushing is always recommended. Brushing different areas of the mouth in the same order every time has been shown to increase brushing effectiveness. Cleaning is optimized by using multiple and overlapping strokes. Pay special attention to those areas most frequently missed when brushing —the most *posterior* (back) molar in all of the arches, the canines (bicuspids), and the *facial* (surface on the cheek side of the tooth) aspects of the *lower anterior* (front) teeth. Be careful to brush correctly or you can cause the teeth to wear away (which may cause them to become sensitive).

Toothpaste

For centuries baking soda or salt have been the classical dentifrices of choice. However, in their pure form, they did not have a palatable taste. Since the 1940s, toothpastes have become more effective and pleasant tasting. In the mid-20th century a new era of therapeutic toothpastes was introduced when an ingredient called *fluoride* was added to toothpaste to fight decay. Until about 1985 all toothpastes were basically the same. They consisted of four ingredients: an abrasive, fluoride, a flavoring, and a foam. However, studies over the last 10 years have indicated that the addition of certain ingredients in toothpastes gives them specific improvements, which marketers focus on in advertisements. Toothpastes have now been formulated to eliminate decay, reduce tartar, freshen breath, whiten teeth, circumvent allergies, eliminate tooth sensitivity, and minimize *aphthous ulcers*. They come in pastes, gels, drops, and powders in every color and flavor imaginable.

Many toothpastes on the market today contain fluoride in varying concentrations and compounds. Studies have determined the advantages of each fluoride compound, but none has been shown to be ideal. There is one toothpaste on the market containing stannous fluoride that advertises it reduces gingivitis. The maker increased the stannous fluoride content to 0.45 percent, which put the level of fluoride high enough to interfere with plaque activity. Tests have shown that with regular use gingivitis and bleeding points are reduced. However, the increased stannous fluoride resulted in greater staining on the teeth.

The "hottest" item on the current toothpaste market is the "plaque preventing" or "plaque inhibiting" toothpaste. These new anti-tartar toothpastes have been successful in reducing *calculus* buildup between scheduled six-month appointments. However, even when they are used regularly, they have not totally eliminated tartar. These toothpastes should be used in conjunction with, not instead of, regular visits to your dentist or his hygienist to have your teeth cleaned. Some dental authorities are concerned that plaque-controlling toothpastes can give the patient a false sense of security. The usual signs and symptoms of periodontal disease are bleeding and swollen gingiva. These toothpastes may prevent the occurrence of these early warning signs; thus, the patient may delay a periodontal evaluation. In short, the periodontal disease may become advanced before it is treated. Therein lies the danger.

Many users have also complained about the unpleasant taste in these dentifrices. Another concern for those using the anti-tartar toothpastes is the tooth sensitivity that sometimes occurs after long-term use. Some patients seem to be sensitive to sodium pyrophosphate, an active ingredient found in some anti-tartar dentifrices.

There are several toothpastes on the market today designed to combat tooth sensitivity, which studies show occurs in about one in seven patients. These dentifrices usually contain potassium nitrate, sodium monofluorophosphate, strontium chloride, or sodium citrate. Tooth sensitivity may be caused by the use of abrasive toothpastes on root surfaces, or it may be a normal response to gingival recession that occurs around an otherwise healthy tooth.

These toothpastes have varying levels of acceptable taste, and they are usually recommended for use in conjunction with office treatments. If you use one of these dentifrices for two or three weeks and your teeth are still sensitive, you need to be sure to tell your dentist. You could have a tooth that needs root canal therapy, or you may have periodontal disease. Delay in dental treatment could mean the loss of one or more teeth.

The foaming agent found in many toothpastes that creates the perception of effective cleaning is sodium lauryl sulfate. At least one study to date has indicated that some patients prone to aphthous ulcers report a significant decrease in ulcerations when this ingredient is removed from the toothpaste.

If you are someone fighting bad breath it might be interesting to note that some toothpastes contain various essential oils that reduce odors. Oxidants such as peroxides neutralize the more noxious odors. Chlorine dioxide, considered one of the most powerful oxidants available today, is found in one of the popular toothpastes on the market. A side benefit of these ingredients is that they improve gingival health.

Until recently, abrasion was the only way to mechanically remove extrinsic stains to create whiter teeth. Fifty percent of the average toothpaste is composed of abrasives. Abrasives, during use, remove cementum and expose the dentin, which is the pathway to the pulp. Too much abrasive action, a problem for about 25 percent of the adult population, can cause teeth to be sensitive. If you are an adult, there are yet other considerations. Adults get dental caries, but their worst enemy is periodontal disease. Periodontal disease means that there is *cementum* and/or *dentin* (tooth structure located below the enamel of the crown of the tooth) exposed to the oral cavity. If the teeth have exposed cementum and/or dentin surfaces, the degree of abrasiveness of the dentifrice used can be a definite consideration.

The toothpastes used to remove tobacco stains are very abrasive. The abrasiveness is what removes the stain from the teeth. But if you have exposed root surfaces, this abrasiveness can make the teeth sensitive. So it's really a trade-off. By using these toothpastes, you can remove tobacco stains, but you may also end up making your teeth sensitive. The frequency of use of these abrasive toothpastes is also a factor that affects the sensitivity of teeth. Consider too, you are at a higher risk for periodontal disease, if you are a smoker.

If you are using chlorhexidine rinses for periodontal therapy you may have already experienced problems with staining on your teeth and restorations. Some toothpastes contain calcium peroxide or citroxain, which helps reduce or prevent chlorhexidine staining.

The good news is that recent evidence shows it is possible to whiten teeth and remove stains without eroding or abrading the tooth structure or restorations. This could create a whole new market in dentifrices.

Any toothpaste you consider should have the ADA Seal. This is the only way to be sure it has been tested for safety and efficacy, and that the claims made by the manufacturer are true.

Dental Floss

Another important aspect of home care is flossing. It removes plaque and food particles from between the teeth and under the gum line where the toothbrush cannot reach. Not removing plaque can lead to decay at the point of contact, and, even worse, results in periodontal disease.

Floss was first commercially introduced in the United States in 1882 by Johnson and Johnson Company of New Brunswick, New Jersey. In the beginning almost all dental floss was made from multiple filaments that were combined into a strand. The more twists per inch the strands were given, the less likely the floss would fray when applied to the tooth surface.

Over the past few years dental floss has really come of age, and shopping for it is like going to an ice cream store: You have all flavors and varieties from which to choose.

You will find: plain, mint, or cinnamon flavor; extra wide, extra fine; shred-resistant; and "super" floss. If that is not enough, most of these come waxed, unwaxed, or lightly waxed. There are also a number of special-purpose flosses that have been developed for the consumer-oriented dental marketplace of the 1990s. These include floss impregnated with fluoride, and looped floss that is composed of standard unwaxed floss on one side of the loop and fluffy blue floss on the other side that can be used to clean teeth and massage the gums.

Then there is the paraphernalia for the real floss junkies. These include manual floss holders, some with adjustable arms and built-in floss holders, a battery-powered flossing device that produces sonic vibrations as the floss head glides up and down in the interproximal spaces, and an acrylic fiber yarn that has a preattached threader designed to floss in wide spaces and under bridges. It is usually easier to floss under bridges when floss holders are used. There is even a power-assisted interdental cleaner on the market. Of course, you can also purchase small spiral or single-tuft interproximal brushes (made of plastic or foam) with detachable handles; softened, wooden, wedge-shaped toothpicks; folded gauze strips to be used by rubbing them back and forth between the teeth; and a toothpick inserted into a plastic handle with contra-angled ends for adaptation to the surfaces of the teeth.

The following are basic instructions for flossing:

1. Cut off about 18 inches of your favorite type, size, and flavor of floss.
2. Wrap about 14 inches around the index finger of one hand.
3. Wrap the rest around the middle finger of the other hand, and use this finger for taking up used floss.
4. With about an inch of floss between them, the thumb and forefinger are used to guide the floss between the teeth.
5. Work the floss between the teeth, using a sawing motion. Never snap the floss: This can result in serious injury to the gingiva.
6. Gently work the floss down the side of the tooth until it meets the gingiva. Then gently slide the floss into the space between the gingiva and the tooth.
7. Curve the floss into a C shape against the surface of the tooth. Move the floss away from the gingiva, using a scraping action along the side of each tooth. Repeat this action four to five times per tooth surface.
8. Repeat steps 2 through 7 with a clean segment of the floss for each tooth.

It may be easier for children to use a loop of floss. To do this, they should take a piece of floss about 10 inches long and tie the ends together into a circle. Then hold the floss tightly between the thumbs and forefingers and proceed. Most children, by age eight, are able to floss their own teeth with parental supervision.

It is important to floss daily, and the best time is often in the evening, perhaps at bedtime. If you do not have good finger dexterity, you may want to use a commercial floss holder.

When flossing, I suggest that you start with the same tooth each time and move clockwise around the mouth until all the teeth have been flossed. The idea is simply not to miss any teeth. In addition, do not forget to floss the back side of each tooth in the upper and lower dental arch.

When you first start using floss, your gingiva may be sore for five or six days. Flossing may even cause the gingiva to bleed. As the plaque is broken up and the bacteria are removed, your gums should heal and the bleeding should stop.

See your dentist if bleeding gingiva persist. This could be a sign of improper flossing technique, which can be harmful. Bleeding gingiva can also be a sign that you have moderate to severe periodontal disease.

Most periodontists surveyed today say that neither waxed or unwaxed floss is better. Just floss! Dr. Sebastian Ciancio, professor and chair of the Department of Periodontics at the University of Buffalo, recently stated in an article that "it's the mechanical action of flossing that reduces plaque and bacteria levels around teeth and gums and is a key for preventing or halting adult tooth loss." Even though it is important, flossing is certainly no substitute for brushing.

Mouthwashes

For many years mouthwashes have been used primarily for cosmetic reasons. Most of the "antiseptic" mint-flavored mouthwashes are quaternary ammonium compounds that contain cetylpyridinium chloride and domiphen bromide. Research shows that these agents can reduce dental plaque and gingivitis, but their main focus is to freshen breath or sweeten the mouth temporarily. They also aid in removing food particles. Experts in the field say that the freshening effects of these mouthwashes last for about 15 to 20 minutes. They do not cure bad breath. And anyway, bad breath is not a disease to be "cured." Bad breath can be caused by everything from the foods we eat to serious oral or general bodily infections. For the most part, mouthwashes only mask breath odors. In most cases, the "antiseptic" mouthwashes do not carry the ADA Seal.

There are several fluoridated mouthwashes available over the counter that have the ADA Seal. The mouthwashes on the market that contain fluoride have therapeutic value because fluoride has been shown effective in reducing tooth decay. The ADA recommends the daily use of a fluoride mouth rinse for those over age six. Most health professionals recommend you take the liquid into your mouth, swish it around vigorously for about a minute, and then spit it out. Do not swallow! For maximum benefit, it is recommended not to eat or drink for 30 minutes after rinsing. Bedtime is generally the best time to be sure the fluoride rinse's action is not disturbed.

There are several antimicrobial mouth rinses on the market today. They are recognized by the dental health professionals as being useful as a preventive agent (anti-plaque and anti-gingivitis), having therapeutic value, and useful in assisting in certain professional procedures.

Listerine was the first over-the-counter anti-plaque and anti-gingivitis rinse to be given the ADA Seal. This antimicrobial mouth rinse is a phenolic agent that contains additives that fight plaque by interfering with its formation and/or by killing plaque bacteria. Some patients experience an initial burning sensation and bitter taste, but accommodation usually occurs in a few days. These mouthwashes should be used as part of your daily preventive home care routine. They are not, however, to be used as a substitute for brushing and flossing.

The therapeutic value of antimicrobial rinses is recognized by health professionals who use them as a preprocedural mouth rinse. The antimicrobial rinses with the ADA Seal have been shown to be so effective in killing bacteria that many dental professionals now have patients use them before dental procedures to prevent the spread of microorganisms during aerosol-generating procedures (e.g. when decay is removed from the tooth with a high-speed hand piece). These mouth rinses have also been shown to be very important to patients who are at risk for bacteremia. Antimicrobial mouth rinses have been recommended as a supplement to antibiotic premedication for patients at risk for bacterial endocarditis. Dental professionals also recommend that patients who have implants, crowns, bridges, and orthodontic appliances use these mouth rinses.

Chlorhexidine (Peridex) is the most widely used member of the bis-biguanide class of broad-spectrum, antimicrobial antiseptics. It is considered useful in treating specific bacterial and fungal diseases. Many dental professionals recognize it as useful for post-oral surgery to help treat patients with hyperplasia, drug-induced dry mouth (xerostomia), and oral infections. It is also recognized as very effective in maintaining plaque control and gingivitis. Unfortunately, it is available only by prescription. It should be noted that chlorhexidine does have disadvantages. It has been shown to cause the following: staining of the teeth, an increase in calculus buildup, dental hypersensitivity, and an alteration in taste sensation. Some dentists have reported they ask patients to dip their toothbrush into some Peridex solution and then brush with it, rather than rinse. This seems to decrease the problem with altered taste, and it allows specific problem areas to be treated. Chlorhexidine is inactivated by most dentifrice surfactants, so it must not be used in proximity with regular toothbrushing. It is recommended that you wait at least 30 minutes after use before your brush your teeth. It does have the ADA Seal.

The anti-plaque, pre-brushing dental rinses come in several flavors (including mint) and a variety of colors. They usually contain sodium benzoate or benzoic acid, which are both antimicrobial. However, many of them do not have the ADA Seal.

The oxygenating agents for reducing mouth odors contain hydrogen peroxide and baking soda. Recent studies reveal that these mouthwashes show promise for reducing plaque and gingivitis, but safety concerns have been raised over the chronic use of peroxide. A very popular mouth rinse in this category does not have the ADA Seal, even though the toothpaste by the same name and manufacturer does carry the Seal.

Studies show that the effect of all of the mouth rinses can be enhanced when delivered in a powered oral irrigator. Traditional mouth rinses deliver the agent about 1 mm below the gum tissue. In contrast, when an irrigating device is used the agent is delivered 3 to 4 mm below the gum tissue.

Name-brand mouthwashes come in several flavors and colors; these are expensive because of the tremendous cost of national advertising. However, supermarket and discount stores copy the composition of the successful name-brand products. Purchasing these can save you money if you know what to look for in buying the house brand.

Some brands of mouth rinses contain from 14 to 27 percent alcohol. Research indicates that nine ounces of mouth rinse with 14 percent alcohol or as little as 4.5 ounces of mouthwash with 27 percent alcohol is a potentially *lethal* dose for a 20-pound child. That is why as of May 1, 1995, the ADA requires all manufacturers who want the ADA Seal to have child-resistant caps on products that contain more than three grams of alcohol. For the convenience of elderly and households without children, one size of the product may be sold without child-proof caps. Sample-size bottles are also not required to have the child-proof closure.

There have been some reported cases of problems with overuse of mouthwash (e.g. burning mouth) due to the alcohol content and change in oral bacteria. Therefore, it should always be used according to directions or as your dentist has directed. More is not always better.

Before you buy a mouth rinse, read the label to be sure you are getting a mouth rinse that fits your needs. Several different categories of mouthwashes have been discussed above, and each one has a specific purpose. And remember, if it has the ADA Seal you can be sure of its safety and effectiveness, and also that the claims by the manufacturer are true.

Toothpicks and Other Periodontal Aids

Toothpicks can be used to clean out food caught between the teeth—but beware. Toothpicks, along with cigarettes, saccharin, and certain children's toys have gained attention as a potential health hazard. That is right: Toothpicks are under attack by both physicians and dentists.

Dr. Lawrence Budnick of the Center for Disease Control and Prevention (CDC) in Atlanta has estimated that over 8,000 toothpick-related accidents occur each year. He adds that this figure might be low.

In a recent article, Budnick reported three toothpick-related deaths. The toothpicks were swallowed, puncturing the stomach and/or intestine, and death occurred.

Children aged five or younger are most frequently severely harmed by toothpicks; eyes and ears are the sites most frequently injured. This kind of injury is 20 times greater in children five or younger than in any other group, but children aged five to fourteen are also at peak risk. There is no doubt about it: Toothpicks should be kept in child-resistant containers.

Of the adult population, those aged 25 to 44 most frequently swallow toothpicks. Alcohol and hors d'oeuvres make a dangerous combination when the hors d'oeuvres are held together by toothpicks. The toothpicks should always be visible. Denture wearers should be especially cautious, as they do not have the ability to "feel" the toothpick. Neither do they have the same ability to discriminate objects being chewed as do non–denture wearers.

Many dentists do not recommend toothpicks for their patients. An alternative is the "soft" toothpick that can be purchased at most pharmacies. It is called the *interdental stimulator*, and you can buy it in a variety of flavors. Though both soft and hard varieties are classed as toothpicks, the difference is that the standard toothpick is made of a harder wood and can splinter, causing gum injuries. The interdental stimulator is made of soft balsa wood, triangularly shaped (to more properly fit the space between the teeth), and does not splinter. If you use the interdental stimulator, moisten it first to make it softer. This will prevent much potential injury. Neither type of toothpick eliminates the need for a good toothbrushing.

To clean between your teeth, the best devices are a soft toothbrush, the rubber stimulator on the end of some toothbrushes, or perhaps, best of all, dental floss.

Oral Irrigating Devices

The ADA states that there "is no substitute for brushing and flossing." However, consumer marketing estimates indicate that about one in six households have *oral irrigating devices.*

Oral irrigating devices, or oral irrigators for short, use water from a reservoir, pump it through a hose, and force the water out of the tip end of the hose. The water jet aids in cleaning debris from between the teeth. You are probably most familiar with the trade name Water Pik, which has become a generic term for all oral irrigators. The original Water Pik was designed by a dentist/mechanical engineer in Fort Collins, Colorado; it has been marketed since 1962 by the Teledyne Corporation.

There are currently several oral irrigators on the market that have been given the ADA Seal. The ADA states that the effects of pulsating and non-pulsating water are equivalent, so this becomes a personal choice when choosing an oral irrigator. The most important thing to remember before purchasing is to be sure the oral irrigator you are considering has the ADA Seal so you can be sure the product is safe and effective, and that the manufacturer's claims are true.

The benefits of oral irrigators include: cleaning around crowns, cleaning under and around bridges; cleaning orthodontic braces; and helping to clean out periodontal pockets. The oral irrigator aids in washing out food particles and bacteria that toothbrushing and flossing miss, but it is not a substitute for either of these.

Several studies have investigated the effects of mouthwashes that contain chlorhexidine, phenolic-related essential oils, and stannous fluoride. They have determined these mouthwashes can be enhanced when delivered in a powered oral irrigator. When compared with rinsing with the product or using plain water in the powered irrigator, these mouth rinses were much more effective. Research has shown that mouth rinsing cannot deliver the mouth rinse more than 1 mm below the gum tissue. However, when mouth rinse is delivered with an oral irrigator, it reaches 3 to 4 mm below the gum tissue.

Not all patients need oral irrigators. Ask your dentist whether he thinks you need one to meet your particular needs. If he feels you do, ask him how to use it to your best advantage.

Some words of caution: The bathroom could be a hazardous place to use an oral irrigator. There is a danger of being electrocuted if the unit falls into water (sink, tub, and toilet) while you are using it. Most of the ADA-certified oral irrigators are encapsulated to prevent accidental shock to its user. However, it has been suggested that permanent wall brackets would minimize or eliminate this potential problem.

The ADA currently issues the following warning: The oral irrigator should not be used if its use causes pain. In addition, the ADA states oral irrigators can force bacteria into your bloodstream. Patients who have heart murmurs, hip replacements, etc. should keep this last statement in mind. You should ask your dentist and physician if there is any question of the oral irrigator's safety in your particular instance.

The oral irrigator should not be used if you have a tooth abscess, severe periodontitis, or a "predisposition" to bacterial infections. One additional warning should be considered. I have personally seen a patient with deep periodontal pockets involving the upper teeth puncture the floor of the nasal sinus by using an oral irrigator. It is suggested by many dentists to use the oral irrigator at its lowest setting to prevent self-induced injuries. High settings could push debris into the tissue rather than pushing it out, as intended. When it comes to these devices, more is not always better.

Some periodontists feel that the real danger of oral irrigators is that the patients like them so well that they neglect their brushing and flossing. As the ADA aptly points out, the irrigator is only an adjunct to brushing and flossing; it is not a substitute. But used correctly, it can be a very good aid in maintaining good oral health.

ASKING QUESTIONS

The most important service you can do for yourself as a dental consumer is to be informed. Be aware of what your dentist is proposing for your treatment. Let us assume that he has told you that you need one "simple" cavity filled. Which tooth is it? How can you prevent any similar cavities from forming? What type of filling is needed? How much will it cost? Ask plenty of questions if you are uncertain of what is going on, or what is about to happen to you. It is your tooth and your mouth, and you have every right to know what is going to happen!

Dental consumerism has just begun to march forward with a force of concerned patients. An excellent example is the impact that 10,000 concerned people in California had when they requested a California Dental Association Dental Patient Bill of Rights! This bill states that patients have the right:

- to see a dentist every time they receive dental treatment
- to know in advance the type and expected cost of treatments
- to expect dental team members to use appropriate infection controls, such as gloves and masks
- to ask about treatment alternatives and be told, in a language they can understand, the advantages and disadvantages of each
- to know the education and training of their dentist and the dental team
- to know what professional rules, laws, and ethics apply to their dentist and the dental team

The California Dental Association has stated that numerous requests for copies of the Bill of Rights have come from all 50 states and 12 foreign countries. The newspaper column Dear Abby and a *Los Angeles Times* editorial praised the California Dental Association for urging patients to exercise their consumer rights.

Informed consent is a very important aspect of dental care today. Patient education about necessary treatment alternatives, or the ramifications of no treatment, should be accomplished at the diagnostic appointments (such as when you go for your routine tooth cleaning and checkup). Economics do sometimes dictate which option you must elect. For example, you might decide on an amalgam (silver filling) rather than a gold onlay. The amalgam may not be the best choice, but it will save the tooth until you can save enough money to select the better choice. Ask what your options and risks are in selecting a particular course of treatment.

Having a thorough understanding of your needs allows you to understand treatment plans *before* treatment is started. For every procedure you need your dentist should inform you about treatment alternatives (advantages and disadvantages), cost, risks, and ramifications of non-treatment.

How do you know whether your dentist is charging you a fair or reasonable fee for his services? That is a tough question to answer. Information to help you make this evaluation can be found in the Dental Fees chapter.

If you have any doubts about the necessity of a restoration, the experience or the expertise of the dentist, or if there is anything else that bothers you, *do not hesitate to speak up.* The dentist cannot read your mind. If the problem is one of confidence in the dentist, do not hesitate to change dentists or at least seek another opinion.

Now, let us assume that you have chosen a dentist, and you need a restoration on your lower left first bicuspid. Do you know which tooth this is? This could be very important information to know later. Why? What if you get a toothache while on vacation? If it is on the left side, you can tell any dentist that you recently had a filling on the lower left first bicuspid, and thus the toothache might be coming from that tooth. You need to be able to communicate with a new dentist who is not familiar with your dental history. It is also helpful to be able to communicate effectively with your regular dentist. It is up to you! In the beginning a toothache is localized. Later the pain becomes diffuse and it may be difficult to determine its source. If you are informed, you could be a great help in the diagnosis. It's also important to know how deep the filling was and whether a pulp capping (sedative medication placed on exposed pulp) was necessary. You could be helping yourself out of an uncomfortable situation later.

In addition to the technical side, you should take into account the human aspects. A big question is: Can you communicate with your dentist? Find another dentist if the answer is a big "No!"

Finally, after you get home, you can examine the treatment done by your dentist. It is quite easy, provided the dentist placed a silver or gold filling. Does it feel as though the filling is hitting first when you bite down? If the answer is "yes," go back and tell your dentist. He can "adjust the occlusion" (fix the bite) by grinding down some of the dental restoration. Watch for tooth sensitivity or sharp pain, which also may indicate a high restoration.

Next, you can purchase a mouth mirror from the dental aids section of your local pharmacy. It will look just like the one that the dentist used except that it will probably be made of plastic rather than metal. There should be no "catch points" on the restoration between the teeth when you floss. It should be smooth; thus, you can use your finger nail to test this and to make sure that you have no obvious open margins (spaces) between the tooth structure and the filling material. An open margin can eventually lead to decay under your restoration.

If there is a question of the quality of the service provided, first bring it to the attention of the dentist who provided that service. If you get no satisfaction, seek the advice of another dentist or your local dental society.

PEER REVIEW: A SOLUTION FOR THE CONSUMER

Dental and medical malpractice cases cost everyone. Malpractice premiums have skyrocketed over the last several years and the cost is still rising. I am sure it does not come as too much of a surprise that these additional overhead costs are passed on to the consumer. That is the way any business works; consumer prices must be increased to offset increases in business expenses.

Big verdicts against dentists are still fairly rare. In fact, according to statistics, 80 percent of the court decisions are in favor of the dentist. The question you should ask before seeking legal advice is: Did the dentist fail to perform to your expectations or was he truly negligent? Maybe you would be ahead in the long run to communicate directly with the dentist to try to resolve the difference of opinion or to go through the peer review process sponsored by your local dental society.

The *peer review* system is an alternative to legal intervention in disputes between dentists and their patients. Every dental society has a peer review system in place to resolve problems that arise between the patient and his dentist. The system involves a special committee of volunteer dentists who agree to consider the questions of the quality and/or appropriateness of the dental care provided. This committee is usually called a peer review committee. You may refer to the address and telephone numbers of state dental associations located in the back of this book to contact the peer review committee in your area.

Members of the peer review committee are trained to deal impartially with cases. In addition, there is never a charge for a peer review judgment. The process is simple so that patients will use it. You are usually asked to write a letter stating the facts of your case and the nature of your complaint. As with correspondence concerning any type of complaint, stick to the facts and leave out name-calling and emotional wording. You want to present yourself as a reasonable person. The committee will then examine the dentist's treatment records. They will talk with you and your dentist separately. The committee might even want to examine you if they feel it would help resolve the issue.

Finally, both you and your dentist will be advised of the recommendation of the peer review committee. Realize in advance that no dentist can be forced to follow the recommendations of the peer review committee. But very few dentists want to appear unreasonable and/or gain a reputation for practicing substandard dentistry. Peer pressure in these cases is very strong if you have a reasonable complaint.

You can only use this system if there is no malpractice litigation pending, so you must initiate action in peer review before you get an attorney involved in the case. Peer review is a simple system that can usually rectify your problem in a swift, objective manner. Since no attorney fees are involved, it certainly could be much more beneficial to you than a long, drawn-out court case.

DENTAL CARE DURING PREGNANCY

Probably at no time in a woman's life do her teeth need more conscientious care than during pregnancy. This will not only help reduce dental disorders that are exaggerated during pregnancy, but it will also insure that the unborn child has good general and dental health. Good oral health is achieved by regular brushing, flossing, eating a balanced diet, and professional checkups.

Studies show most pregnant women experience *pregnancy gingivitis*, a condition that causes red, inflamed, and bleeding gingiva (gums) during pregnancy. It occurs because dental plaque, a bacterial build-up associated with tooth decay, accumulates on the teeth and irritates the gingiva. It occurs more frequently during pregnancy because there is an increased level of hormones in a pregnant woman's body. The higher level of hormones exaggerates the way the gum tissue reacts to the irritants in plaque. It is important to note it is still the plaque, not the increased hormone level, that is the major cause of gum disease. Keeping your teeth particularly clean during pregnancy, especially near the gum line, will help dramatically to reduce or even prevent gingivitis during pregnancy.

One myth I have heard mothers repeat is that during pregnancy their teeth get "soft" and are more prone to decay. What really happens is these mothers get pregnancy gingivitis. Since the decay process begins with plaque, their teeth are more susceptible to decay. It is normal for pregnant women to want to snack frequently between meals, which in turn exposes their teeth to repeated acid attacks on the tooth enamel. Many people do not realize that each time they eat, acid attacks the tooth enamel for at least 20 minutes. The increased hormone levels of a pregnant woman cause plaque to become more of a gum irritant. This is a really good reason to be particularly concerned about keeping your teeth brushed with a fluoride and plaque retardent toothpaste and flossed.

Concern for your child's teeth should begin when he/she is still in the womb. Your baby's teeth begin development as early as six weeks into the pregnancy and start to calcify between the third and sixth month of pregnancy. These developing teeth need vitamins A, C, and D, minerals, calcium, and phosphorus. Expectant mothers have a responsibility not only to their own health but also to the health of their unborn baby. If you are an expectant mother, you should be aware of the special needs of both your own and your child's teeth. This means you need to eat the right foods. The simpliest way to assure good nutrition is to eat a well-balanced diet, with foods from each of the four major food groups. These major food groups are: bread and cereal; fruits and vegetables; dairy products; and meat or fish. The recommended diet for pregnant women usually includes three servings of dairy products, two to three servings of meat, poultry, or fish, six or more servings of breads, grains, or cereals, three or more servings of vegetables, and at least two servings of fruit.

Food cravings frequently include sugary snacks. Soft, sticky, sweet foods such as cakes, candies, and dried fruit are especially harmful because they stick to the teeth, which prolongs the acid attack. Substitute for sweets more wholesome foods such as cheese, fresh fruits, or vegetables. They are better for your teeth and provide more of the nutrients your baby needs.

Another myth believed by many people is that calcium is lost from the mother's teeth during pregnancy. This is not true. The calcium your baby needs comes from your diet, not your teeth. It is true, however, that if your calcium intake is inadequate your body will provide this mineral by taking it from your bones. Since the primary source of calcium is either dairy products or supplements it is important for you to consult with your physician to be sure you are getting enough calcium during pregnancy.

It is best to schedule your dental visit during the fourth to sixth month of pregnancy. Be sure to let your dentist know you are pregnant when you see him for your regular checkup (which should not be neglected because of pregnancy). Most dentists include a question about pregnancy on their health history forms. If it is necessary to see him for an emergency be sure to let him know you are pregnant when you call to make the appointment. Many dentists will want to consult with your physician before any treatment is started. Stress, past miscarriages, or the use of certain drugs can all have an influence on the approach and timing your dentist chooses to take in attending to your dental needs.

The first three months of pregnancy are thought to be of greatest importance in the unborn child's development. For this reason, X rays, dental anesthetics, pain medications, and antibiotics are usually not prescribed during the first trimester, unless absolutely necessary. Most antibiotics, pain medications, and anesthetics come with a standard warning that the drug should not be used during pregnancy without the advice of a physician. Women who could possibly be pregnant or who are in early pregnancy should consider this fact carefully before taking such a drug.

The antibiotic tetracycline is of special concern to pregnant mothers. Normally it is safe and effective, but it comes with the following warning: Tetracyclines should not be used by expectant mothers, especially during the last half of pregnancy. They should not be used by nursing mothers. And they should not be prescribed to children age eight or younger. In the expectant mother, these antibiotics can retard the developing baby's bone growth. Studies show tetracycline can also cause discoloration ranging from yellow to gray to brown in the crown (the visible part of the tooth) as it develops.

If you have any doubts or concerns, insist that your dentist and physician discuss your particular needs. If you are given a prescription by your dentist, *do not exceed the prescribed dosage.* This includes the use of aspirin.

Dental X rays, if necessary, are much safer today. The exposure time is very short with high-speed film, and the body can be protected from scatter radiation by using a lead apron with a thyroid collar. If your dentist has *digital imaging radiovisiography* (RVG) he can take X rays using about 90 percent less than the usual radiation exposure.

During the last three months of pregnancy, the stress associated with dental visits can increase the incidence of certain prenatal complications. In addition, sitting for an extended time in the dental chair can be especially uncomfortable during the last three months.

The administration of dietary fluoride supplements to pregnant women cannot be recommended because there is no conclusive evidence that it reduces dental caries in the teeth of their offspring. The ADA does recommend that fluoride supplements be started on children six months after birth. The reason is that the crowns of all the primary teeth and the crowns of the permanent incisors and first molars have begun their development. It is important for these teeth to receive exposure to systemic fluoride during their early development.

At the time of your dental visit, realize that pregnant women may be more prone to gagging than before. Do not be alarmed. It is perfectly normal, and dentists are aware of this situation.

Parents are a role model for their children's behavior and their dental health. As a parent, you need to become familiar with good dental practices. This includes appropriate pacifiers, proper oral hygiene for infants and young children, the use of fluoride, and regular dental visits for your child (which should begin before one year of age).

2

General Dentistry: The Backbone of Dentistry

I feel that it is important for the consumer to have an understanding of the background of the basic training of the general dentist (generalist) upon graduation from dental school. The profile of the average dental school applicant is three to four years of college credits prior to dental school admission. The pre-dental program includes liberal arts, science, and math requirements.

Dental school training usually lasts four years. During those four years, the first year is devoted to the academic aspects of dentistry and basic sciences as they apply to dentistry. The second year is a continuation of the first year plus numerous laboratory courses that are preparatory to providing patient treatment starting the next year. During the third year, treatment provided by these students is under direct supervision of dental school faculty. The fourth and final year of dental school is devoted to completing minimal clinical (patient treatment) requirements in each of the ADA-recognized specialty areas. Finally, after passing a National Board exam, every dentist must pass a state or regional board exam for each state in which he wants to get a license to practice dentistry.

In summary, the general dentist has a college background and then completes four years of dental school. He has a broad background in all areas of dentistry and can legally perform any treatment permitted in dentistry in which he feels competent. The general dentist, however, has an ethical and legal obligation to refer, or at least confer, with a dental specialist when he has any question about the diagnosis or treatment of a patient or when that treatment is beyond the scope of his training and experience.

THE OTHER TEAM MEMBERS

Dentists in the past often worked alone or with a single office assistant. Now a dental assistant can complete a one-year, ADA-approved training program if he wants to become a registered dental assistant (RDA). These assistants are then eligible to take a Dental Assisting National Board Certification Examination to become a certified dental assistant (CDA). Anyone who is trained on the job or who graduates from a nonaccredited program must first work two years before taking the CDA exam.

A dental hygienist is required to complete a two-year, ADA-approved training program before becoming a registered dental hygienist (RDH), and only then is he eligible for licensure. He must pass a state board exam for each state in which he wants to get a license to practice dental hygiene. University-based hygiene programs may offer a bauccalaureate, and sometimes a master's degree, if the applicant completes at least two more years of schooling.

Today we have a "dental team" rather than the single practitioner. This provides more efficient delivery of dental care. Even the duties of the assistant and hygienist are expanding, partly because of advanced training. Thus, the term "expanded duties" has come into the vocabulary of the dental profession. This means that assistants and hygienists are performing tasks previously the sole responsibility of dentists. The dentist has indirect responsibility for the actions of personnel under his direction, regardless of their training and experience.

Even though there is overlap with several specialty areas, the "bread and butter" of the practice of the general dentist is called *restorative dentistry* because he is restoring teeth. The general dentist's practice also places emphasis on the preventive aspects of dentistry at the "grassroots" level. Hygienists are directly involved in this aspect of a dentist's practice. This includes periodic checkups with an oral exam, X rays, and dental *prophylaxis* (teeth cleaning).

In your visits to his office, your dentist and/or his hygienist should stress the importance of good oral hygiene. This involves not only having your teeth cleaned at his office on a regular basis, but also practicing good oral hygiene at home.

About half of the dental offices in this country employ a dental hygienist. The hygienist works in close contact with the dentist and the other office staff to provide full and economical services to dental patients. For you as a consumer of dental care, the hygienist is a well-trained member of the dental team who provides a multitude of services for the dentist and the patient. Their functions include: teeth cleaning, teaching the patient home care (brushing and flossing), and nutritional counseling, and in some states with special training, they may even administer dental anesthesia.

The American Dental Hygiene Association (ADHA) reports that only about 2 percent of the hygienists in this country are men. Most of the male hygienists that are currently licensed were introduced to the field in the military service.

DENTAL X RAYS

X rays are a very important part of your oral exam. They are taken to disclose a number of problems that cannot be seen in other ways. These include damage to jawbones caused by *periodontitis*; early signs of *orthodontic* problems in children; *impacted* teeth; abscesses, cysts, or tumors in the jaws; and injury from trauma to the teeth caused by being hit or falling. The biggest reason for having X rays, however, is for early detection of decay between the teeth. Detecting a problem early rather than treating it after it has become painful saves patients time, effort, and expense.

The dentist is the best judge of when X rays should be taken. Each of us has different health needs, so the frequency of X-ray exams has to be individualized. The schedule for needing radiographs at recall visits varies according to your age, risks of disease, and signs and symptoms. Children may need X-ray exams more often than adults because their teeth and gums are still developing and their teeth are more likely to be affected by dental caries. X rays may be required before, during, or after dental treatment. It is a good idea to have copies of appropriate X rays sent to your new dentist if you change dentists or are being treated by two dentists (perhaps a general dentist and a dental specialist) simultaneously. It will help in the diagnosis of current problems, and save you the expense and needless radiation exposure of getting another set of X rays.

There is no doubt that dental X rays are useful, but many times patients are uncertain about their level of risk to exposure to them. Most dental professionals agree the level of radiation exposure from a full-mouth series (usually about 16 films) is about the same as either a day spent outside or spending the weekend sitting in front of a color television. Thus, dental X rays are a definite benefit with risks that are not much more dangerous than the risks inherent in everyday living.

Pregnant women are usually advised not to have X rays unless absolutely necessary. Remember, however, that dental X rays are now safer than ever before. X-ray equipment is carefully regulated to comply with standards established by the U.S. Public Health Service. The ADA cautions that dental films "should not be taken before the dentist has examined a patient and determined whether they are needed."

For your protection, modern dental offices have safeguards to help minimize any potential risk of X rays. These include: high-speed film that can cut the exposure time in half (the use of digital imaging radiovisiography cuts the exposure time by 90 percent); filters to eliminate unnecessary X-ray exposure; devices to limit the size of the X-ray beam to a small area; shielded, open-ended X-ray cones that limit scattered radiation; and precise timers to provide consistent exposures.

In addition, the ADA recommends the use of lead aprons for X-ray examinations to eliminate any unnecessary exposure. The lead apron protects the reproductive organs from exposure to radiation.

One additional note is in order about lead aprons. The lead apron that your dentist uses on you should have a thyroid collar to protect your thyroid gland from unnecessary radiation. Studies on the subject have found two major reasons for this extra protection. First, the thyroid gland is very susceptible to the uptake of radiation. Second, the thyroid gland is directly in line with the X-ray beam of some of the projections your dentist takes in doing a full-mouth, X-ray exam.

It is likely that in the near future we will be able to eliminate further potential hazards from X rays. In the early 1980s dental researchers at the University of California at Los Angeles (UCLA) began working on a technique called *dental xeroradiography*. This technique has been useful in medicine for some time; it has been routinely used in breast X-ray examination. Xeroradiography gives excellent contrasts between shades of black and white on an X-ray film, thus providing better diagnostic films with lower radiation-dose exposures than you would be subjected to by traditional X-ray films used in most dental offices today.

Now in the 1990s a new technique called digital imaging radiovisiography is being perfected. This revolutionary technology has three major benefits for dentists: it enhances patient understanding of treatment, minimizes time spent on developing X rays, and dramatically reduces the amount of patient exposure to radiation. Digital imaging radiovisiography is the direct replacement of X-ray film with a sensor (an electronic image receptor) linked to a computer. Instead of capturing the image on an emulsion, an electronic chip called a CCD (charge coupled device) is used. The CCD is also used in video cameras. The sensitivity of the receptors and the digital nature of the image permits the patient's X-ray dose to be reduced by 80 to 90 percent of that needed by conventional film, depending on the system used.

The *intraoral camera* also uses a sensor to capture the image of the outside surfaces of the teeth and tissue in the patient's mouth. Instead of being a replacement for the X ray, it allows the dentist to move around the patients mouth and have the images instantaneously appear on the computer screen. The dentist is able to show the patient large areas of decay in the teeth, broken or leaking restorations, questionable pathology, and otherwise invisible cracks in symptomatic teeth.

The CCD technology was adapted for use in intraoral cameras and digital imaging radiovisiography. Both of these technologies share the same underlying operating principles. Computers are used to store the images, to enchance the images with color contrast and zoom capabilities for more accurate and precise diagnosis (magnification from 100 to 300 percent), to duplicate the images, and to transmit the images via modem to an insurance company or to another dentist for an instant consultation. Both of these systems can be networked with business management or voice-activated periodontal and restorative charting software. The system enables patients to see an image instantaneously on a monitor, and this allows them to interact and communicate easily with the dentist and his staff. This broader area of information technology is expected to reengineer the practice of dentistry over the next 10 to 20 years. These technologies are not improvements over existing systems. This is a breakthrough! At this time about 57 percent of the dentists in the United States are using intraoral cameras but only 1 percent have digital imaging. As the cost decreases and the technology is improved, more dentists are projected to have this technology available in their offices.

Now let us examine the use, types, and limitations of the traditional X-ray films that your dentist takes in doing his oral examination. When X rays pass through your mouth, the more dense body parts (such as healthy teeth and bone) absorb more X rays than the soft tissues (such as the cheeks, gums, and/or diseased bone or teeth) before striking the film. This creates a contrasting image on the film.

The dentist will take a *periapical X ray* when he wants to see the entire tooth from crown to root apex. The periapical film gives the dentist information on: the presence of dental caries, the depth of fillings, the presence or absence of insulating bases under existing fillings, the possible presence of any bone loss at the root apex which might indicate an infected root canal, and any internal or external resorption of the tooth root.

Most dentists feel that a *full-mouth survey* is necessary every two to three years. Usually, fourteen periapical and four bitewing films (two on either side of the mouth) make up the full-mouth survey. *Bitewing* X rays show only the crowns of the teeth. They give the best view of caries between teeth, the pulp chamber, and how close the filling and/or insulating base is to the pulp. Bitewing films are usually taken on those visits to the dentist when a full-mouth survey is not yet indicated. This subjects you to minimal X-ray exposure while allowing the dentist to find dental caries while it is small.

To insure a thorough diagnosis, most dental authorities recommend a panoramic radiograph be taken at least every five years. A *panoramic radiograph* is one large, single X-ray film that shows the dentist all structures in the lower half of your face. The film is exposed by a special X-ray unit in which the X-ray tube automatically moves around the patient's face.

Panoramic radiographs allow the dentist to see: the sinuses, bones in the cheeks, jaw fractures, possible tumors in the lower half of the face, "extra" teeth, "hidden" impacted teeth (those not erupted and located far from their proper location in the bone), and sometimes teeth needing root canal therapy.

Other special types of X rays are taken by your orthodontist. These will be discussed further in the chapter on orthodontics.

As an aware dental consumer, you should be knowledgable of the limitations of dental X rays. It is very important to realize that interpretation of the dental X ray always relies on subjective judgment. Studies have shown that when several dentists examine the same X-ray films to determine if dental caries is present and needs to be treated, the dentists are lucky if they agree 75 percent of the time.

Recently, there was a study done on endodontically treated patients. Patients were evaluated at a two-year recall to determine if the bone loss at the root apex had resolved. There was about a 40 percent disagreement among the authorities, who were dental specialists!

This does not mean that dentists are incompetent, it simply illustrates that the criteria for both dental caries and healing of bony infections are quite difficult to define. The difficulty arises because these matters are subject to individual interpretation.

You may be wondering by now what an X-ray film does demonstrate. It is a shadow of a three dimensional object. The film can only show differences in the degree of calcification in a tooth or bone. Most studies tell us that there must be at least a 40 percent loss of mineral from a mineralized tissue such as bone or tooth before the dentist can see the pathology on an X ray. That means that by basing all the diagnosis on X-ray examination, the dentist could miss many important pathologies. He will simply not see the pathology unless there is enough demineralization for it to appear on an X-ray film. It takes several X-ray films over a period of time to make a determination of progressive pathology. But lack of X-ray film findings is no reason to go through life with a painful toothache. Sometimes intervention must be based upon symptoms.

Dental X-ray films are indeed important. In addition to determining dental decay, X rays can be used to detect oral cancers.

RESTORATIVE DENTISTRY

In the past 30 years remarkable changes have occurred in restorative dentistry. The changes are related to factors that include: an aging population that is retaining their natural teeth and experiencing frequent decay on root surfaces, reduced decay in children because of access to fluoride, the availability of new and better restorative materials, increased demand for esthetic procedures, and better materials for bonding to tooth structure. Current technology has forced dentists, dental schools, and dental examining boards to make significant changes.

Restorative dentistry includes all aspects of restoring fractured, missing, or decayed teeth. Teeth, as described in chapter 1, are composed of several dental "tissues": enamel, dentin, cementum, and pulp. When one or more of these tissues becomes defective, it is necessary to restore the tooth to its normal function. Hence, the term "restorative dentistry."

Restorative dentistry, which is the bulk of the treatment a general dentist performs, encompasses several procedures with the particular choice depending on both the extent and the cost of the repair. The types of restorations a general dentist does include: *amalgams, inlays, onlays, composite resins* (tooth-colored fillings), and *crowns* (gold, porcelain fused to metal, and porcelain).

As a general rule of thumb, it can be said that the larger a restoration the more likely it will have to be restored with a crown. Tooth-colored restorations are most commonly used in anterior teeth, although some dentists now use them in posterior (back) teeth. Abscessed teeth need to have root canal therapy before they are restored. It is usually mandatory that a crown be placed on posterior teeth that have had root canal therapy. Teeth that have been badly broken down many times need to be reinforced with a post (a small metal rod) cemented in the canal before a crown is cemented on the tooth. It is important to remember that *no* restoration (silver or gold) is "permanent."

Let us now examine the specifics of how the dentist accomplishes restoration of your teeth back to function. In addition, let us examine what options you have.

43
▲

Silver Fillings . . . and Mercury

One of the most common materials used to restore teeth that have tooth structure destroyed by decay is *amalgam* (a filling material that contains alloys of mercury, silver, copper, tin, and sometimes zinc). Dental restorations using amalgams are an inexpensive and durable way to restore teeth that are amenable to this type of restoration. The metal mercury is added to the alloy, and, when mixed, the mass created is pliable for a short period of time. This material is placed in small increments into the tooth structure from which the dentist has removed the decay. The mass of amalgam is built up to extend beyond the normal anatomical contour of the tooth. Then the excess amalgam is carved away until the tooth is restored to its original contour prior to the destruction caused by the dental decay. Amalgams are durable, less expensive than gold, have the ability to withstand the intense pressures of chewing, and are easy to place and replace.

Dental amalgam restorations can be found in the majority of people's mouths in the United States. Ninety percent of the dentists in North America still use this method. A recent survey concluded the longevity of amalgam restorations decreased as the restoration size increased. For example, single-surface amalgams last about 13.5 years, two- or three-surface amalgams average 9.7 years, and larger four- or five-surface fillings last an average of 6.1 years. Many authorities now feel the practice of re- placing amalgams because of defective margins should be reexamined with consideration given to the caries-risk status of each patient, since marginal breakdown may merely indicate the restoration is aging and not necessarily that there is caries present. Other authorities feel that decay progresses very slowly in many patients, and if caries is present in these patients and it has not progressed past the enamel, it should be treated with fluoride to remineralize (harden) the enamel and monitored.

The question of the safety of dental amalgam has been studied for over a century. Since the early 1980s it has been a controversial issue in this country due largely to a group led by a dentist in Colorado that made claims linking mercury to a number of medical problems. Recently the state attorney general, on behalf of the Colorado Board of Dental Examiners, filed a complaint that led to this dentist losing his license. The complaint notes the dentist was censured by the state board in 1983 and given 18 months probation, with continuing education requirements and practice restrictions.

According to the ADA there is no valid, scientific evidence that associates the minute amount of mercury vapor in dental amalgams with any health problems. For more than 100 years studies have been conducted worldwide on dental amalgam in tooth restorations, and no link has ever been found between these amalgam restorations and any medical disorder. Mercury is found in food, water, and air. There is always a very low level of it present in our bodies. The daily dose of mercury from these non-dental sources exceeds the amount released from dental amalgam fillings. The Food and Drug Administration has concluded that amalgam causes no demonstrated clinical harm to patients, and removing amalgam fillings will not prevent adverse health effects or reverse the course of existing disease.

Over the last few years *amalgam bonding* has become popular. This technique requires an extra step. Instead of putting the amalgam directly into the prepared tooth, a layer of resin is put in first. The resin bonds to the tooth, and the amalgam bonds to the resin. This type of restoration reduces tooth sensitivity and is stronger than a traditional amalgam restoration. Many authorities consider it the state of the art procedure for amalgam fillings. Mercury-free metallic materials that are currently being developed also show promise. However, as the demand for esthetic fillings increases, many authorities predict amalgam will be phased out.

Only a very small number of people are sensitive (or allergic) to mercury. A mercury allergy can only be determined by an allergist or related specialist. It is usually manifested as a simple skin rash. This tiny group of people (less than 1% of the population) should avoid amalgam restorations. Your dentist can advise you if you are found to be sensitive to dental amalgam.

Amalgam restorations are held in place by mechanical retention. In other words, amalgams do not "stick" to tooth structure. You need adequate tooth structure remaining to "hold" the restoration in place. In lieu of adequate supporting tooth structure, grooves, dentin bonding agents, or a combination of both can sometimes be used to retain the amalgam in the tooth cavity. Dentin bonding agents that adhere to dentin and materials such as amalgam and composite resins (tooth-colored fillings) have been developed to replace tooth structure and give extra strength. An added benefit is that they seal the dentin tubules, preventing sensitivity. If there is not enough remaining tooth structure, full-coverage crowns with internal support (i.e. *posts*) may be your only option.

If you elect to have an amalgam restoration, ask your dentist about the difference in cost and durability between silver and cast metal or porcelain restorations for the same tooth.

Past studies have shown that the average silver restoration lasts many years before it needs to be replaced. Today's newer amalgams are expected to last even longer. Dentistry is continuing to provide better services with its ongoing research. This research includes both protecting you from harmful materials and improving restorative materials.

Gold Fillings (Inlays and Onlays)

If your dentist has told you that you need a gold filling you might think immediately about a relative or friend who has a gold crown (cap) that covers the entire outer surface of the crown of the tooth. You probably thought that was what you were going to get. Wrong! A gold filling (inlay or onlay) restores a cavity in the tooth from which the decay has been removed. It does not, however, cover the entire tooth, like a crown does when it is placed. In discussing gold fillings, basically, you have two options: an inlay or an onlay.

Knowing the advantages and disadvantages in these types of restorations will make you a wiser consumer.

INLAYS AND ONLAYS

Both inlays and onlays are custom-made restorations that are made (cast), using gold and alloys, from a mold of your tooth. These two types of fillings require less tooth structure be destroyed when the tooth is prepared than crowns, and they are more esthetic because the part of the tooth that shows when a person smiles is left intact. This also means there is never a problem with matching because the natural tooth left is nature's perfect match. These restorations usually require two visits. At the first visit the tooth is prepared and an impression is taken. A temporary covering (filling) is usually placed to protect the tooth. The impression is usually sent to a lab so the restoration can be created using the model of the patient's tooth. This insures the restoration will fit precisely in the tooth. In the next visit the dentist checks to be sure the custom-made restoration fits perfectly, and it is then cemented in place. A more detailed discussion of this process can be found under crowns in the Prosthodontics chapter.

Custom-made restorations are made either of a combination of metals called alloys, or of porcelain. *Alloys* contain precious metals such as gold and palladium or non-precious metals such as chromium, tin, copper, and sometimes nickel or zinc. *Porcelain* is a natural looking restoration made of a very strong glass. It is possible to blend the different colors of porcelain to get an exact match of the adjacent teeth where the restoration is being placed.

Inlays are designed to fit within the contours of the tooth. The reason to restore a tooth with an inlay is that the tooth is usually so badly destroyed by caries (decay) that an amalgam is difficult to keep in the tooth. Unlike an amalgam which is held in the tooth strictly by mechanical retention, a gold inlay is cemented. Even though most modern compositions of dental amalgam come very close to the strength provided by gold, gold is usually considered a better choice provided the price is not beyond your means.

It is important to notice I have used the words "placed" and "cemented." *No inlay should be pounded or beaten into place!* This will split the tooth because it causes the inlay to act as a wedge. Since you can split a log using the mechanical advantage of a wedge, think of the fragile tooth. For this reason, it is crucial to have an inlay placed only by a highly competent (and careful) dentist. A properly placed inlay, prior to cementation, should fit extremely closely to the remaining tooth structure without the dentist having to exert any forces to place it in the tooth. In other words, it should not be placed using excessive force. In addition, the *margins* (the point where the tooth structure and the metal meet), should be smooth . . . there should be no "catch points" when you or the dentist go across this junction with any fine instrument. And the point of contact between the inlay and the adjacent tooth should be loose enough to allow dental floss between the teeth but not so loose as to allow food to pack between the adjacent teeth. Lastly, the inlaid tooth should not be high in occlusion (bite). In other words, when you're biting on the inlaid tooth it should *not* hit before the rest of the teeth. The bite should be even on all teeth. High or premature occlusion could injure the pulp or most certainly the bony support of the tooth. Injury to the bony support and *periodontal ligament* usually causes the tooth to be sensitive or sore when you bite on it.

Though an inlay and an onlay are very similar, an *onlay* always covers some or all chewing surfaces of the tooth. An onlay binds together and protects the tooth's *cusps* (the pointed elevations of a back tooth). In my opinion, a gold onlay is the better of the above two restorations.

All of the points concerning inlays (having good margins, good contact points with adjacent teeth, and good retention) also pertain to onlays or any other dental restoration. Two other points should be kept in mind about onlays. First, the design of the cavity preparation differs from an inlay because with an onlay the cusps are cut down on the natural tooth so that they may be replaced (covered) by gold. The gold lays over or "onlays" the cusps. A properly placed onlay, just as with an inlay, should not be pounded into place. This could cause a cracked tooth, which has a very poor long-term life expectancy.

Second, discuss the cost, durability, and retention of the proposed onlay with your dentist. Sometimes a gold crown (three-quarter crown, veneered crown, porcelain or porcelain-fused-to-metal crown) could save you time, money, and possibly the tooth itself in the long run at a slightly greater cost. These different types of crowns will be discussed and described in the chapter on prosthodontics.

New technology has brought dentistry several versions of the *computer-aided design/computer-aided manufacture* (CAD/CAM) systems.

These free-standing, cart-based systems enable the dentist to design and fabricate dental restorations at chairside without using conventional methods for making inlays, onlays, veneers, crowns, and bridges.

The systems are comprised of the following components:

1. a camera with a precision optical system
2. a monitor to view and manipulate the image of the tooth
3. design software and a keyboard for drawing construction lines to enable the restorations to be precision designed for each individual case
4. a milling chamber to fabricate the restorations after they are designed

The systems utilize blocks of ceramic restorative material in various shades and sizes. After the tooth is prepared and the rubber dam is placed, contrast powder is applied to the isolated area and an optical impression is taken with the camera. The image then appears on the monitor and the doctor outlines the contour of the preparation. His outline will be reproduced as a restoration when the system has completed the milling process on the block of ceramic restorative material. After checking to be sure the restoration is correct, it is then seated and polymerized (cured). The edges of the restoration are then finished and contoured by the dentist. The advantages of using these systems are:

1. conservative tooth-colored restorations can be fabricated without having to remove unnecessary tooth structure
2. the restorations can be fabricated in just a few hours because no outside lab is needed

The fees for these restorations are usually higher than lab-fabricated restorations because the technology is so new and so few dentists in the U.S. have the systems. Many authorities feel the concept has great potential, but at this time the systems are very expensive and there is some room for improvement in the marginal integrity (fit) of the final restorations.

Tooth-Colored Fillings

Technology today has answered the call for more esthetic restorations. More attractive than gold or silver, tooth-colored fillings are, as the name suggests, fillings that match the natural color of your teeth.

Decades ago the first tooth-colored fillings were called *silicates*. Today we have newer and better materials. Tooth-colored fillings are available in two categories: composite resins and glass ionomers. These materials have literally revolutionized the field of esthetic dentistry.

Composite resins are plastic materials made of glass and resin. Today virtually all of them are photo-cured (hardened) with visible light. They are used both as fillings and to repair defects in the teeth. Malformed or misshapen teeth can be recontoured to a more pleasing appearance. These materials can even restore the tooth to about 85 percent of its natural strength because they literally stick the tooth together. Because these fillings are tooth-colored they are difficult to distinguish from natural tooth structure.

Composites are typically used in front teeth where a natural appearance is important. Their use in back (posterior) teeth is limited. However, in the last 20 years posterior composite resins have improved substantially in the area of color matching, wear resistance, and marginal integrity. Authorities are still concerned about their durability when exposed to the pressures of chewing. They do not last as long as silver fillings. Studies also indicate there is shrinkage when they are cured (hardened under light), which can lead to recurrent decay in susceptible individuals. If they fracture they have to be replaced because it is not possible to repair them. There are several composite resin filling materials available that are ADA approved, and most of them are marketed for use on both anterior and posterior teeth. At this writing many authorities feel posterior composite resins remain technique-sensitive and difficult to place. They are also more complicated than silver fillings because they require several extra steps not needed with amalgams. Not all patients are good candidates for this material because they must maintain a very high level of oral hygiene.

Glass ionomers are tooth-colored materials made of fine glass powders that are used to restore teeth, particularly on exposed root surfaces where the gums have receded. The roots of teeth are covered with dentin (a softer tissue than enamel) so they are more prone to decay when exposed. Glass ionomers contain fluoride, which is slowly released to help prevent further decay in these receded areas.

Bonding and Bleaching

With the emphasis in today's society on a healthy appearance and an attractive smile, bleaching has become a safe way to enable patients to have bright, white teeth. A recent survey indicated 60 percent of general dentists are providing tooth bleaching procedures in their office, and 85 percent are dispensing take-home bleaching agents to their patients. Studies show 50 percent of all people want to have whiter teeth. Staining occurs on the surface of teeth when they are exposed to tobacco, certain foods and beverages (e.g. coffee, tea, and berries), and by accumulation of tartar deposits and calculus. Internal discoloration sometimes occurs in teeth when too much fluoride is present in the water, when teeth are traumatized, or if the antibiotic tetracycline has been taken during the time teeth were forming. Discoloration is also very obvious when silver amalgam restorations are placed in the anterior (front) teeth. The two most current methods of correcting tooth discolorations are bonding and bleaching.

BONDING

Bonding is yet another method to enable the dentist to repair, to protect, or to return a discolored tooth to its natural color. It is also commonly used to close gaps between front teeth, repair chips, protect exposed roots that result from gum recession, and restore teeth after decay has been removed. It is the latest in "esthetic" dentistry. There are two basic techniques for bonding. One technique, which is called *direct bonding*, is performed directly in the mouth in one appointment. The other technique, which is called *indirect bonding*, is a two step indirect process.

Direct bonding involves the following:

1. The tooth is slightly reduced (contoured) on the front side to prevent the "new" tooth from being too bulky. This does not usually require the use of anesthesia.
2. The tooth is acid-etched, washed, and dried.
3. A composite resin, the same type of tooth-colored material that is used to restore teeth (see chapter 2), is applied to the surface of the tooth, contoured into the proper shape, and allowed to harden using a special light or chemical process. The tooth is then smoothed and polished.

Now the esthetically "repaired" tooth appears natural. Sometimes it is necessary to come back for a follow-up appointment for final polishing and finishing. This technique has been used by dentists for about 20 years. The new bonding materials are almost as strong as natural tooth structure. They can be expected to last at least five years before they have to be replaced. You can help maintain your bonding for a longer period of time if you do the following:

1. Avoid acids (tomatoes, pineapples, and vinegar) and alcohol. These items will damage the resin material.
2. Avoid items such as cigarettes, tea, coffee, or berries because they will stain the resin material.

3. Do not eat ice, popcorn kernels, or hard candy because it might cause excess pressure on the bonding material.

The indirect bonding technique incorporates the use of custom-made shells (*laminated veneers*) that are affixed directly to the tooth, usually without the need for anesthesia. These veneers are similar to fingernails that are contoured and bonded over your existing nails. They are made of composite resins, acrylic, or porcelain. Many authorities feel the porcelain ceramic veneers are preferred because of their longevity, resistance to surface discoloration, reduced bacterial adhesion, and superior esthetics. They are, however, more expensive.

The steps are as follows:

1. The tooth is reduced to insure that the laminated veneer will contour properly when it is bonded on the tooth. Otherwise, it will look and feel bulky.
2. An impression of the tooth is taken and sent to the lab where the veneer is made to match the color and shape of your teeth.
3. The tooth is prepared by roughening the front surface with mild etching solution. The laminated veneer is then bonded on the tooth using a composite resin cement.

In order to avoid discoloration, it is usually recommended that patients with veneers avoid coffee, tea, tobacco, red wine, and other pigmented foods (e.g. cherries and blueberries). Veneers can chip and peel off so patients must avoid habits such as chewing on hard objects (e.g. ice, nuts) and fingernail biting. A realistic expectation for this technique is three to twelve years before it must be replaced.

BLEACHING

Bleaching natural teeth under the supervision of a dentist is both safe and effective. When patients use over-the-counter products that are not recommended by their dentist, many times they find out these products can irritate soft tissue. Some of the recent over-the-counter (OTC) bleaching kits use acetic or citric acid as their active ingredient, which causes major structural damage to enamel and dentin. This results in tooth sensitivity and gingival irritation when used for an extended time. These ingredients may also have a detrimental effect on tooth filling materials. The trays in the over-the-counter bleaching kits are not custom-made, resulting in leakage of the bleaching agent on the tissue in the mouth.

Bleaching supervised by a dentist can either be done in the dental office or at home. Your dentist is able to bleach both vital and non-vital teeth. A *vital tooth* is one that has a healthy pulp. A *non-vital tooth* is one that has had the pulp removed by root canal therapy.

When bleaching is done in the office on vital teeth, it takes from 30 minutes to one hour per visit. In order to protect the soft tissue, a gel-like substance is first applied to the gums and then a rubber shield is used to cover the gum tissue, allowing just the teeth to be exposed. A solution of an oxidizing (bleaching) agent is then applied to the teeth, and a special light is focused for 20 to 30 seconds at five-minute intervals. This helps activate the oxidizing agent. The process usually needs to be repeated several times before the tooth is the desired color. As of this writing, the only bleaching agent to receive the ADA Seal of Approval for dentist-supervised office use is Starbrite Bleaching Solution by Stardent Laboratories.

Bleaching that is done at home should also be supervised by your dentist to insure no damage occurs to your teeth or gums. Nightguard vital bleaching (NGVB) with a 10 to 15 percent carbamide peroxide has replaced most techniques for bleaching multiple teeth that are vital (have not had root canal therapy) at home. This technique, when done under the supervision of a dentist, is painless, inexpensive, and very effective. Most authorities favor the thicker gels that are flavored. The gels are easier to handle if they are dispersed in syringes instead of bottles. Before the bleaching technique can begin, your dentist has to make you a custom-fitted nightguard out of thin, soft materials that will minimize the potential for temporomandibular joint (TMJ) problems, tooth sensitivity, tissue irritation, and orthodontic problems. This appliance will cover all of the upper or the lower teeth. First, an impression of your mouth is taken. Then a custom-made nightguard is fabricated with reservoirs to hold the bleaching agent in place. The nightguard is designed to fit closely over the teeth in order to prevent excessive loss of the bleaching agent. This also prevents the tissue from being injured by coming into contact with the bleaching agent. The fee for the above described vital bleaching ranges from $150 to $350 per arch. In contrast, when a dentist bleaches in the office the charge is per treatment. It is very important for patients to return on a scheduled basis to the dentist to have him check the progress of the treatment and the condition of the gums and teeth.

Before bleaching is started at home, the patient needs to brush his teeth and clean his mouth thoroughly. Then, after a thin rope of gel has been placed in the nightguard, the guard should be inserted in the mouth. There should be enough gel in the nightguard to cover the teeth without overflowing on the gum tissue. Most home bleaching products recommend three to five minutes' exposure to a maximum of two times each day. You need to consult your dentist for his recommendation on the amount of treatment exposure you should have each day and the best times for you to do the treatment. It is generally recommended that the treatment should not continue more than six weeks. No documented studies have assessed the longevity of vital bleaching, but the general feeling is that patients will eventually need re-bleaching.

Bleaching should be stopped if teeth become sensitive, allergic reactions manifest, severe discoloration occurs, caries is present, or if the patient lacks motivation to follow directions properly. Tooth sensitivity usually subsides if the patient skips a day or if fluoride (provided by the dentist) is used in the tray instead of bleach for that night. Results, which are not always predictable, have been reported to be better with teeth that have a yellow-orange discoloration. Overall, more than 90 percent of the patients treated in this manner have reported some degree of success.

Non-vital bleaching is performed on teeth that have had root canal therapy. These teeth are bleached from both inside and outside the tooth. Studies have shown this is a more predictable procedure because the bleaching process is not limited to the enamel of the tooth's crown. First, the involved teeth are isolated with a rubber dam, and then a portion of the filling material in the tooth (usually gutta-percha) is removed. Next, a temporary cement is placed inside the tooth to prevent the bleaching agent from entering the remaining filled canals of the tooth. After the cement sets, a thick mixture of the bleaching agent (usually sodium perborate and distilled water) is placed in the open cavity. The mixture is then packed tightly and the hole in the tooth is covered with cement. The mixture is usually renewed at two week intervals. The number of renewal sessions is determined by the type of staining and how well it responds to bleaching. When satisfactory results are achieved, the cavity is cleaned out and then filled with a tooth-colored restorative material.

A major advantage of bleaching over other procedures that whiten teeth is that it doesn't require any tooth structure to be removed. It is usually recommended that teeth be bleached a shade lighter than you desire, since they will darken with time.

Pulp Capping (Direct or Indirect)

Dental decay or caries usually first attacks the tooth somewhere in the enamel of the crown. The caries progresses deeper with time. As soon as it reaches the dentin, the caries causes irritation of the dental pulp. Remember, the dentin is the pathway to the pulp. You, as a patient, sense there is something wrong with the tooth at this point because you may have sensitivity to cold, hot, sweets, or just breathing in air. The sensitivity may be spontaneous (having no apparent cause), transient, or prolonged.

The source of your pain is the dental pulp. If the pulp is inflamed to the point where it will not recover or the pulp tissue is dead, the pulp may have to be removed through root canal therapy or endodontic treatment. But if the inflammation has not progressed this far, then the dentist may be able to preserve the pulp through pulp capping. Essentially, this procedure involves cleaning out the decay and then placing a protective base over the exposed area.

There are two types of pulp capping—direct and indirect. In *indirect pulp capping*, the decay is removed down to the softened dentin. That is the extent of the cavity preparation. A *base* made from various compounds and cements is placed over this remaining softened dentin. Bases not only protect the pulp from discomfort produced by thermal changes but also protect the tooth from irritation of the restorative materials. The theory is that the softened dentin is not infected and will *remineralize* (harden) under the base.

In *direct pulp capping*, however, the dentist cleans out all the decay and soft dentin, thus exposing the pulp. Another type of base is placed over the pulpal exposure site. Using this technique, the dentist does not leave softened dentin under your final restoration. The base is supposed to create a mineralized bridge over the exposure site an thus "heal over" the area. The success rate for direct pulp capping seems to be higher than for indirect pulp capping. Direct pulp capping succeeds about 85 to 90 percent of the time, depending on the study quoted, whereas indirect pulp capping works about 70 percent of the time. If either procedure fails, root canal therapy will be necessary.

The controversy with pulp capping is whether the fate of this tooth should rest on a pulp capping, which has a less certain future than root canal therapy. Many dentists today prefer to go ahead with the root canal therapy and play the safer odds. Realize, if the pulp capping fails, you will know it from either an X-ray exam and/or painful symptoms which could include a full-blown abscess. Any tooth with pulp capping should be monitored by your dentist for continued pulp health by a regular examination, including periodic X rays.

ANESTHETIC AGENTS

An anesthetic is the chemical substance that the dentist injects into your oral tissue to produce pain-free dental treatment for you. The first local anesthetic to be isolated and studied was cocaine. In the early 1800s it was noted by physicians that it was used by the ancient Peruvians to alleviate hunger, relieve fatigue, and uplift the spirit. In 1884 the Viennese physician Dr. Karl Koller introduced cocaine into clinical medicine as an anesthetic. Koller had learned about cocaine from another Viennese physician, Dr. Sigmund Freud. This popular anesthetic was soon found to have major concerns, including addictive qualities and potential toxicity.

The concerns about cocaine's lack of safety led to the development of the second generation of anesthetics (the ester types), which resulted in the discovery of procaine. Shortly afterward three more ester-type anesthetics were synthetized: propoxycaine, tetracaine, and chloroprocaine. However, these anesthetics were found to have a propensity for evoking allergic reactions in a clinical application.

This led to the development of a third generation of anesthetics (the amides), which are popularly used today. Lidocaine, an amide-type anesthetic, was first synthetized in 1943, and is today considered the "gold standard" against which all other local anesthetics are measured. The most common anesthetics injected by dentists today are either Xylocaine (lidocaine) or Carbocaine (mepivacaine), another amide anesthetic. The first name is the trade name and the second name is the generic name.

Xylocaine comes in a 2-percent solution with either 1:100,000 or 1:50,000 parts of epinephrine, a vasoconstrictor. A *vasoconstrictor* is an important component of most anesthetics that serves two functions. First, it partly shuts down the blood circulation in the area. This helps in surgery because there is less bleeding in the area to be surgically treated. Its other function is to keep the area anesthetized longer since a smaller volume of circulating blood allows the anesthetic to remain at the site for a longer period of time. This reduces the likelihood of any toxic reaction because the anesthetic is removed very slowly from the needed area. Thus, less anesthetic is needed to keep the area anesthetized. The safety record with Xylocaine is superb, although some allergic reactions have been reported. It is important for patients to realize that epinephrine can cause heart palpatations, but this is not the same as an allergic reaction to the anesthetic. Our bodies produce their own epinephrine, and palpatations can be a result of anxiety. Xylocaine starts working anywhere from instantly to four minutes after injection. The anesthesia lasts about two and a half hours in most patients.

Carbocaine is the second most commonly used anesthetic. Carbocaine comes in either a two-percent or three-percent concentration without any epinephrine. Because of the lack of epinephrine, many cardiologists suggest this particular anesthetic be used in patients who have heart problems or are diabetic. Carbocaine's action is such that it will remain in the operative site for up to about 40 minutes without the hazards of adding epinephrine to the solution. It works as fast and as effectively as Xylocaine. *If you are a pregnant mother check with your physician before having any anesthetic administered.* Most physicians would prefer that pregnant women wait past the first trimester (three months) before having any dental injections. If there is any doubt, consult with your physician. But the maximum safe dose of Carbocaine is about half that of Xylocaine.

No drug or anesthetic is without any possible side reactions or allergies. The medical community terms this "risks versus benefits." The use of anesthetics, in most patients, has risks; but these are far outweighed by the benefits.

There are four general principles concerning dental anesthetics administered prior to dental treatment.

1. All anesthetics should be used in the lowest required dose that will provide adequate anesthesia.
2. No anesthetic is without risk in patients who have anesthetic allergies or are seriously ill. Anesthetic allergy reactions have been reported in patients who previously have been administered the same anesthetic without any adverse reaction. However, this occurs only rarely.
3. No anesthetic should be administered by any practitioner who does not have proper emergency equipment and drugs available in case you have a reaction to the anesthetic. There is no guarantee that you will not be the victim of a drug reaction. Rapid, informed intervention could save your life. Make sure your dentist has the proper emergency equipment available.
4. No anesthetic is approved by drug manufacturers for injection into pregnant patients during the first three months of pregnancy. Some anesthetics are not approved for use at any time during pregnancy, and some are not recommended for children prior to their reaching puberty. When in doubt, talk it over with both your dentist and your physician.

Newer Anesthetics

Xylocaine and Carbocaine are not the only anesthetics used by dentists. However, they are the primary anesthetics used today. There are newer anesthetics available that have advantages over Xylocaine and Carbocaine, and the list grows each year. Please understand that the anesthetics discussed in this section are certainly not inclusive of all the new anesthetics.

Now, let us more closely examine the newer anesthetics you might encounter. As previously described, Carbocaine (or mepivacaine) may be administered in a two-percent or three-percent solution without epinephrine (the most commonly used vasoconstrictor). This is now also available in a two-percent solution with a vasoconstrictor called Neo-cobefrin or Levonordefrin (1:20,000).

Neo-cobefrin increases the duration of anesthesia up to one to two and a half hours in the upper jaw and two and a half to five and a half hours in the lower jaw. Contrast these figures to 20 minutes in the upper jaw and 40 minutes in the lower jaw when the Neo-cobefrin is omitted. The onset of anesthesia ranges, in both instances, from thirty seconds to four minutes.

Carbocaine containing Neo-cobefrin has many of the same concerns as anesthetics containing epinephrine. Caution should be used in injecting patients with Carbocaine containing Neo-cobefrin if the patient has a history of high blood pressure, heart disease, or diabetes.

Marcaine (bupivacaine) is used in a 0.5-percent solution. It usually contains 1:200,000 parts of epinephrine. It is chemically related to Xylocaine, rapid in onset of anesthesia, and long in duration of anesthetic action.

Marcaine takes two to ten minutes to produce anesthesia. The anesthesia lasts two to three times longer than Xylocaine. In fact, the duration of the anesthesia has been reported to last up to seven to eight hours!

Marcaine's anesthetic action seems to persist after the numbness has apparently gone. This means that fewer and milder analgesics (or pain relievers) are required postoperatively.

Marcaine comes with and without methylparaben. Methylparaben is the ingredient that acts as an anesthetic preservative. It has been traced to some anesthetic allergic reactions, so many of the newer anesthetics are using another ingredient as their preservative.

Marcaine is especially cardiotoxic (able to bring about a cardiovascular collapse) when used in high doses. This danger is especially real if the anesthetic is inadvertently injected into a blood vessel.

Finally, the manufacturers suggest that not enough research has been done with using Marcaine in children under 12 years of age. An obvious problem is the prolonged anesthetic effect. Children could accidently create severe lacerations of the lip and tongue by chewing their tissues under anesthesia. Children are not responsible enough to be expected not to injure themselves when there is loss of sensation.

Citanest (prilocaine) is a four-percent solution used in many offices for patients who cannot tolerate the epinephrine in most anesthetics. The onset of action takes one to two minutes, and the anesthesia lasts about an hour or slightly longer in some cases.

The manufacturer recommends that Citanest not be used in infected areas or in children under the age of 10. In addition, patients with liver damage or patients who are severely ill should not have the anesthetic used on them. Since Citanest is metabolized by the liver, liver damage can be a contraindication to its use.

All the anesthetics discussed above are safe and reliable when used with proper precautions. All medicines have inherent risks along with their potential benefits. Proper use requires a full health history disclosure, as you can see from the above discussion. When in doubt, discuss your concerns with your dentist and/or physician.

New Approaches to Dental Injections

Dental injections are high on the list of fears we have about going to the dentist. Fear of dental injections has two major aspects. They are: Will the injection keep me pain-free during the procedure, and will it hurt when the injection is administered?

Let us examine both components of the fear of dental injections. Recent research has indicated that one patient in seven experiences some discomfort during dental treatment. Poor anesthesia can occur if the dental anesthetic is not properly administered. Some special techniques to achieve proper anesthesia will be discussed later in this section. These special techniques relieve only the pain of the procedure. The pain of getting the injection can be virtually eliminated using recently developed techniques. There are four major methods used to control the pain of the injection. First, there are relaxation techniques. In addition, there are visualization techniques similar to those used with surgical procedures. These will be discussed in the section on dental fear in chapter 11.

Second, a tropical anesthetic can be used. *Topical anesthetics* range from jellies to ointments applied to the oral tissue in the area to be injected. Some topical anesthetics are sprayed on the tissue. Others are swabbed on the tissue with a cotton swab. Topical anesthetics, which usually contain varying concentrations of Xylocaine or Benzocaine, provide some anesthesia to the surface tissue to be injected.

Third, the dentist may use some distraction techniques. Some dentists gently "shake" your cheek to distract you from the sensation of the injection. Another distraction technique involves the dentist using pressure anesthesia (created by pressing firmly on the spot in the mouth where the anesthesia is to be administered prior to and during the injection). The dentist may use either a finger or an instrument handle to cause pressure. Patients can distract themselves by thinking about other things.

Fourth, the injection is less painful if the anesthetic is warmed to about the body's temperature. The anesthetic solutions can be warmed by special anesthetic warmers, which your dentist can purchase. But a simpler method is to run warm water over the anesthetic carpule prior to injecting its contents. In either case, cool anesthetic solutions seem to produce more discomfort than when that same solution is warmed.

The injection can still be uncomfortable if the anesthetic is not injected slowly. Otherwise, the tissues are distended, causing pain because the anesthesia spreads the tissue apart too quickly. Slow injections allow more solution to be absorbed into the surrounding tissues; thus, less pain is created.

I will briefly discuss some injection techniques. In general, there is infiltration anesthesia and block anesthesia. *Infiltration anesthesia* anesthetizes a specific area of tissue or a specific tooth. *Block anesthesia* anesthetizes a nerve that supplies a certain area of the mouth. Infiltration anesthesia is usually used in the upper jaw, while block anesthesia is usually used in the lower jaw. It is block anesthesia that makes your lower lip, cheek, and part of your tongue numb when you have a lower tooth treated.

Currently, there are some different techniques being used by some dentists to make the certainty of a pain-free procedure more predictable. Some of these are actually rediscoveries of techniques used in the past. Their value has only recently been fully realized.

First, there is a *periodontal ligament injection*. Until recently this technique was used as a supplemental injection when all else failed. In the past, a standard dental injection syringe was used to deliver the anesthetic solution into the periodontal ligament space. Since it takes so much pressure to inject anesthetic into such a small space, a new pressure-type anesthetic syringe has been developed that makes the technique easier to administer and more predictable. Many current articles have recently appeared in the professional literature indicating that the periodontal ligament injection can be used as the sole method of administering anesthetic. Everything from root canal therapy to extractions have been done using the technique (not to mention fillings, crown preparations, etc.). Both effective and safe, it is now possible to anesthetize a tooth in the lower jaw using this method exclusively. This eliminates the need to have the usual extensive numbing associated with the block injection, as previously discussed.

Second, another technique now being used to relieve discomfort during root canal therapy (see chapter 3) is the *intrapulpal injection*. A small-gauge (diameter) needle is used to inject anesthetic solution directly into the sensitive pulp tissue. If the injection is given in two phases, it will be a more comfortable experience. The anesthetic should be injected slowly at first to minimize the discomfort. Then the anesthetic must be injected with pressure into the tissue. You do feel some initial discomfort, but it quickly dissipates.

A third technique, the *Gow-Gates injection*, was invented by Australian George Gow-Gates in 1973. Basically, this injection blocks the major nerve trunk that supplies the lower jaw. The theory is that there are some unusual pathways for the nerves that supply the lower jaw that block anesthesia may not anesthetize. Hence, the Gow-Gates technique anesthetizes the entire nerve trunk to the area. Gow-Gates advocates the use of prilocaine without a vasoconstrictor for the injection.

Another way in which your dentist can provide a more comfortable injection is by using a 30-gauge needle, which is smaller than the 25-gauge needle popularly used in the past.

Some dentists use audio-video analgesia. These dentists use either a wall-mounted television set or special "television glasses," either of which allows you to distract yourself with your favorite program or video games. You might even bring your personal stereo with headphones and turn on your favorite station or recording to whatever volume you might want. Many dentists have found distractions so effective that they routinely use music through stereo headphones to drown out the sound of the drill. This technique sets a pleasant mood and assists in allaying the patient's fears.

Finally, the newest approach to pain control during dental treatment is a technique called *electronic dental anesthesia* (EDA). It involves placing electrodes in the mouth in the area to be treated. The patient uses a hand-held dial to control the amount of targeted pain-blocking signal that penetrates the tissue around the receptor at the treatment site. The benefits of this noninvasive technique (no needles are used) are that it eliminates postoperative numbness, is chemical free, and produces post-treatment analgesia (pain control) because it stimulates the body's natural endorphins and serotonin.

Researchers at the University of Southern California report an 85 to 90 percent success rate for EDA studies that involve amalgams (fillings) and crowns. At this time there are definite limitations to the unit for other types of dental procedures. For this reason the technique has not gained widespread popularity among clinicians. It is contraindicated for use in the following groups of patients: epileptics, patients with chronic circulatory problems, those with pacemakers, pregnant patients, or those unable to cooperate (small children or the mentally handicapped).

PART II

The Dental Specialties

D entistry began meeting the challenge of the new technology explosion several decades ago by creating special areas of expertise called specialities. Specialists take over from general dentists when there are dental problems that are either difficult to diagnose or that require the expertise of someone with extra training in a particular area of dentistry to treat them properly. Sometimes, it may be you who makes the decision to see a specialist; you may want a second opinion or feel that you have special needs. Or your general dentist may refer you to a specialist in certain situations. In fact, the general dentist has an ethical and, perhaps, even a legal obligation to refer patients who have dental problems requiring the skills and knowledge of a specialist.

Unless you specify that you would like a certain procedure to be performed by a specialist, it is up to your general dentist to decide which treatment or treatments should be referred to the specialist. With few exceptions, most specialists want and need to work closely with a general dentist.

Your general dentist is responsible for planning the treatment of each of his patients and must certainly coordinate the services of specialists with his own prescribed treatment. He is ultimately responsible for being sure that all your dental needs are fulfilled.

The American Dental Association currently recognizes eight areas of specialty in dentistry. They are as follows:

endodontist   A specialist concerned with the prevention, diagnosis, and treatment of disorders of the dental pulp and tissues at the end of the tooth root. This includes root canal therapy.

oral and maxillofacial surgeon   A surgical specialist who often performs extractions and reconstructive surgery.

oral pathologist   Among other tasks, this specialist is concerned with the microscopic interpretation, and hence, diagnosis of oral diseases such as tumors and cancers.

orthodontist   A specialist concerned primarily with the correction of maloccluded (crooked) teeth.

pediatric dentist (pedodontist)   A dentist specializing in comprehensive care of children, adolescents, and for special patients who have mental, physical, or emotional problems.

periodontist   A dentist specializing in the *gingiva* (gums) and the bones that support the teeth.

prosthodontist   A specialist who constructs permanent or removable appliances to replace missing teeth.

public health   This dentist usually works for the United States Public Health Service and is concerned with national and international health care planning. Many also work and teach on a communitywide level.

Dental specialists receive an additional two to four years of training in an ADA-approved program in their specialty area after dental school. Their practices are then limited to treatment in their particular specialty area. After they have completed their specialty training they are eligible to take examinations that allow them to become board-certified *diplomates* in their area of specialty. This title gives other general dentists and specialists a measurable way to judge the expertise of the specialist. It also gives the consumer an insight into how the specialist is regarded by his peers.

The function of any specialty area, either in dentistry or medicine, is twofold. First, the specialist should provide better service to patients. No general dentist can know all the information it would take to be a specialist in all areas of dentistry. Secondly, the dental specialties serve as a spawning ground for new information. Specialists have an obligation to add to the base of information available to the profession as a whole. New techniques and/or materials are continually being researched in laboratories and in clinics to determine their safety and efficacy. These investigations are usually performed by specialists. And it is the responsibility of the dental specialist to aid the general dentist in keeping abreast of the most recent developments. Specialists perform this service by providing newsletters, journal articles, and continuing education courses in new methods of treating dental disease to other specialists and general dentists.

Although dental specialists are experts in their respective fields, you may be surprised to discover that their fees are usually comparable with those of general dentists providing the same service.

3

Endodontics

ndodontics is that branch of dentistry concerned with the prevention, diagnosis, and treatment of disorders of the dental *pulp* (soft inner tissues of the tooth) and the tissues at the root *apex* (end). A specialist in endodontics is called an endodontist. A board-eligible endodontic specialist must complete a two-year, ADA-approved training program beyond dental school. Endodontists are experienced in treating complicated cases. They specialize in diagnosing and relieving oral pain and in treating traumatic injuries to the teeth. Their specialty program includes advanced training in performing *root canal therapy* (a procedure that involves removing the pulp of the tooth and cleaning, shaping, and filling the remaining space), and bleaching discolored teeth to make them match the existing teeth. In addition to his expertise on the pulp, the endodontist is also concerned with diseases at the apex of the tooth which may or may not be caused by diseases of the pulp, as well as with the tissues surrounding the roots of the teeth (the *periradicular tissues*). The endodontist uses his advanced training in endodontic surgery to treat many of these problems.

Endodontic surgical procedures include: an *apicoectomy* (surgical removal of diseased tissues resulting from pulpal pathology); *replantation* of teeth that have been accidentally knocked out or intentionally removed and then replaced (or replanted) after surgery has been performed on the tooth apex; a *hemisection* (removal of a root and part of the crown of a multi-rooted tooth); a *root amputation* (removal of a root of a multi-rooted tooth); and *endodontic implants* (utilizing an existing tooth by placing a metal post down the root canal of the tooth and extending into the bone). These procedures will be discussed in succeeding sections of this chapter.

Endodontists are experts in *pulp capping* (see chapter 2). They are concerned with performing a *pulpotomy* (the partial removal of the pulp) when it is necessary to perform emergency relief of pain in adults. In addition, endodontists are adept in performing a *pulpectomy* (locating and removing the entire dental pulp). This procedure is necessary prior to the completion of root canal therapy.

In order for endodontics to be considered successful, the following prerequisites must occur. There should be no *periapical* (around the apex) bone loss if there was none prior to treatment. And if periapical bone loss was present prior to treatment, new bone should regenerate within one to two years after root canal therapy is completed. The method most relied upon to determine success or failure of root canal therapy is to compare recall X-ray films with those taken prior to the endodontic therapy. It takes at least six months for any changes to be visible on an X ray.

Both endodontists and general practitioners who perform root canal therapy are attempting to save a tooth that otherwise would be doomed to extraction. But before starting treatment, one should have realistic expectations of what endodontics can do to save teeth.

Most endodontists view endodontic root canal therapy as a procedure that involves two phases. The first phase is the primary root canal therapy. If problems persist after root canal therapy has been performed, it may be necessary to perform the second phase of the procedure—endodontic surgery. If neither of these approaches prove successful, the tooth may need to either be retreated (the primary root canal filling material is removed, the canals are cleaned, shaped, and then filled again) or extracted. The anticipated rate of success of primary root canal therapy is 90 to 95 percent, unless there are complications of the usual treatment. Retreatment has been shown to have a success rate of about 85 percent at the end of 10 years. Let it be understood that no medical or dental procedure is guaranteed to be 100 percent successful.

Having root canal therapy done today is no longer the bad experience that it was even a decade ago. Root canal therapy should be no more painful during or after the procedure than a routine filling. New anesthetics and anesthetic techniques make most root canal treatments virtually pain free. After the treatment is completed, mild analgesics (aspirin, Tylenol, Advil, etc.) will control over 95 percent of all postoperative pain, which usually only lasts three to four days. Ice packs on the outside of your face and warm saltwater rinses are very helpful in reducing any discomfort immediately after treatment. Again, root canal therapy is done in an attempt to save a tooth that would otherwise be doomed to extraction.

A toothache is many times the beginning sign that root canal therapy is necessary. Let's take a look now at the causes of the typical toothache and what root canal therapy can do to alleviate it.

TOOTHACHE:
ITS CAUSES AND CURES

The management of oral health is to a large extent the management of inflammation. Most people, at some time in their lives, experience a toothache. For some, a toothache is the only thing that will get them into their dentist's office. As a dental consumer, you should know about the major causes and cures of a toothache.

There are two aspects to a toothache: what you can do for yourself, and what your dentist can do for you. When toothaches occur on vacations and in the middle of the night, it may be difficult to see your dentist immediately. You never know when a little self-help can make the quality of your life somewhat better.

The origin of your toothache can be as simple as food trapped between the teeth, which then irritates the gingiva (gums). This situation can be corrected in two ways. First, rinse your mouth vigorously with warm water to remove the debris. Second, you can use dental floss to remove any trapped food or foreign matter from between your teeth.

In the above instance, the problem is with the gingiva and the supporting tissue, not the tooth itself. Usually, with gingival irritation, the pain is low grade, and the tooth is sore to biting forces. Gingival problems can also result in hot and/or cold sensitivity, which can be accompanied by discomfort upon biting. These latter symptoms usually do not occur until the situation is rather severe.

If you are experiencing momentary sensitivity to hot or cold foods it usually is not a signal that you have a serious problem. The sensitivity may be caused by a loose filling or by minimal gum recession that has exposed small areas of the root surface. The symptoms can be eliminated by having the tooth restored and by using toothpastes for sensitive teeth.

A dull ache and pressure in the upper teeth and jaw can indicate sinus problems. The pain becomes particularly intense when the head is bent forward. The pain of a sinus headache is often felt in the face and teeth. Usually over-the-counter sinus and analgesic medications (Tylenol, aspirin) take care of the problem. If the pain is severe and chronic you should see your physician or endodontist for an evaluation. It should be noted that *bruxism* (grinding your teeth, usually at night) can also cause this type of ache. Your dentist should be consulted if you have this problem.

That brings up the next type of toothache: pain from pulpal irritation that manifests as a sharp pain when biting down on food. This delicate tissue of the pulp can be irritated from a deep cavity or a fracture. If you are experiencing a lingering pain after eating hot or cold foods, or constant and severe pain and pressure in the head and neck area, it probably means the pulp has been damaged by deep decay or physical trauma. If you have these symptoms you should have your tooth evaluated by an endodontist to determine if you need root canal therapy. The pulp of a tooth can be either diseased or injured, and be degenerating (or even dead) for some time *before* symptoms occur. In fact, the pulp can be dying and not even the dentist, who is trying to repair the injured and aching tooth, can be sure of the pulpal status until pain occurs. Abscesses do not show up on X-ray films until the infection in the tooth has eroded a "hole" in the bone around the tooth apex (end of root). This usually takes quite a long time to occur.

The pulp is almost certainly "irreversibly" injured if you have pain, especially when accompanied by swelling. In other words, it will not get better! You need to see your dentist and/or be referred to an endodontist immediately so you can get antibiotics to help get the infection under control before root canal therapy can be performed. Pain caused by pulpal injury is more intense and often arises for no apparent reason. If you have swelling, use cold compresses on the outside of the cheek. That brings up two things you should not do if you have visible swelling from an infection in your tooth. First, do not use heat on the outside of the cheek. This makes the problem worse. Second, do not place an aspirin on the gingival tissue of the aching tooth. This causes a severe aspirin burn on the gingiva that only adds to the problem. If you need an aspirin for the toothache, just swallow it; that is where it will possibly do some good.

Pain and/or swelling are not the only indicators that root canal therapy is necessary to save a tooth. On occasion, the pulp tissue will die and the patient will not even be aware of it. Dentists have no way of telling how much insult any given pulp will take. No one knows for sure why some pulps die "quiet deaths." The only sign that a pulp has died may be bone destruction at the root apex. This is determined by a dental X-ray film and other tests your dentist can perform.

Root canal therapy is one highly effective way of treating a tooth that aches because of pulp problems. However, if it is not performed you will have to have the tooth extracted to get rid of the infection.

ROOT CANAL THERAPY

Root canal therapy involves removing the *pulp* (the soft tissue that contains nerves, blood vessels, and connective tissue) and cleaning, shaping, filling, and sealing the canal of the tooth. The tiny dental pulp sometimes gets infected or damaged. The pulp frequently becomes

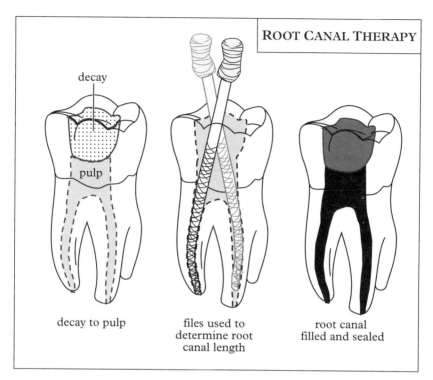

ROOT CANAL THERAPY

decay

pulp

decay to pulp

files used to
determine root
canal length

root canal
filled and sealed

Figure 5

infected because caries (tooth decay) has attacked the enamel, entered into the dentin, and, finally, irreversibly inflamed or killed the pulp. The diseased or dead pulp will, if left in the pulp canal, result in a dental abscess. Byproducts of the diseased pulp can injure the bone that anchors your tooth in the jaw.

You have two options if you have a tooth that is well on its way to becoming a swollen, aching abscess. You can either have the tooth removed (have an extraction) and a replacement (bridge, implant), or you can save the tooth by having root canal therapy and a final restoration placed on the tooth. Saving the tooth also saves you money because it usually costs more to extract and replace a tooth than to treat it by removing the diseased pulp.

Root canal therapy is not exclusively performed by endodontists. In fact, most root canal therapy is performed by general dentists. The endodontist is usually called in by the general dentist when some aspect of the case needs special skills or knowledge.

The person treating your tooth (either the general dentist or the endodontist) will basically follow the steps below when performing root canal therapy on your tooth:

1. A thorough exam, including an X ray, is done to be sure that the correct tooth is being treated. In addition, any complicating factors can usually be seen on the X-ray picture of the tooth prior to treatment. Teeth requiring root canal therapy usually have lingering hot and/or cold sensitivity; sharp, spontaneous pain; often swelling; and sometimes evidence of bone destruction at the apex of the tooth. Any one or more of the above symptoms may be present.

2. After the proper tooth is determined, that tooth is anesthetized by using a local anesthetic. Oral or inhalation sedatives can be given if you feel extremely apprehensive. Most patients do not require any sedation since modern techniques should enable the treatment to be completed with very slight to no discomfort.

3. The tooth is then isolated with a *rubber dam* (a thin rubber sheet about six inches square that is stretched over a frame). In most instances, the rubber dam is used to isolate a single tooth. The rubber dam allows the tooth to be treated in a clean and dry environment. Perhaps as importantly, the rubber dam prevents instruments and medicines used to treat the root canal from being swallowed or inhaled.

4. An access opening is made through the crown of the tooth. This opening gives direct visibility to the canals in the floor of the pulp chamber.

5. The pulp (the soft tissue that contains the blood vessels, nerves, and connective tissues) is then removed from the tooth by tiny instruments called *endodontic files*. Files may be made of either stainless steel or nickel-titanium alloy. These endodontic files clean and shape the root canals to allow them to be filled with an inert filling material.

6. The dentist fills and seals the canal after they have been adequately cleaned and shaped. This prevents bacteria from growing in the canal and causing reinfection. The most universally accepted method of filling root canals among endodontists in the United States is by using the rubberlike substance *gutta-percha*. It is sealed with a cement called a *sealer*. Thus, the bulk of the canal is filled with small pieces of gutta-percha that have been tightly compacted. *Any modifications of this method suggested by your dentist should be discussed with an endodontist in your area before you allow treatment to begin.*

There are a few dentists who still use paraformaldehyde-containing endodontic filling materials or sealers frequently known as *Sargenti pastes, N-2,* or *RC-2B. An April 1991 position statement from the American Association of Endodontists states these materials should not be used for endodontic therapy because they are unsafe.* The document also states "Extensive scientific research has proven unequivocally that paraformaldehyde-containing filling materials and sealers can cause irreversible damage to tissues near the root canal system including the following: destruction of connective tissue and bone, intractable pain, paresthesia and dysthesia of the mandibular nerve, and chronic infections of the maxillary sinus. Moreover, scientific evidence has demonstrated that the damage from paraformaldehyde-containing filling materials and sealers is not necessarily confined to tissues near the root canal. The active ingredients of these filling materials and sealers have been found to travel throughout the body and have been shown to infiltrate the blood, lymph nodes, adrenal glands, kidney, spleen, liver, and brain." The paper further states "the American Association of Endodontists recommends against the use of paraformaldehyde-containing filling materials or sealers because the use of such is below the standard of care for endodontic therapy."

7. X rays usually are taken to determine that the canal(s) are filled to the proper length. According to most endodontic authorities, the ideal point to fill the root canal is one to two millimeters within (or just short of) the root apex. Over 20 research studies have shown that overfilling the root canals lowers the success rate of root canal therapy by 10 to 15 percent. However, this is a calculated risk that can happen to the best dentist. You should not become overly concerned about an overfilled canal in your root canal treatment because your success rate is still 80 percent to 85 percent, which is quite high.

8. Within three months after your root canal is completed, your general dentist should place a final restoration on the root canal–treated tooth. Posterior (back) teeth are usually restored with a crown ("cap") to protect them from possible fracture. A crown may not be required on a front tooth. It is important to refrain from chewing on the tooth until the final restoration has been placed.

Root canal therapy on a tooth can be done in one, two, or more appointments. The more severe the infection and/or the more difficult the case, the greater the number of appointments necessary to complete the case. Let us assume that the case is done in two or more appointments. In that instance, a medication is sometimes put on a cotton pellet, which is then placed inside the tooth to help eliminate bacteria and prevent further spread of infection. Then the access opening, with the cotton pellet, is sealed, using a temporary filling to protect the pulp canal from contamination between appointments. A temporary filling may not be placed if the infection in the bone continues to drain through the root canal as the dentist works to clean out any pulpal remnants. If this occurs, you may be prescribed an antibiotic to control the infection in and around the tooth and bone.

You may feel some degree of discomfort either between root canal therapy appointments or after the root canal therapy is completed. This is to be expected. The dental injections and all the manipulations outside and inside the tooth add to the tooth's soreness to biting forces. You will usually experience a sore tooth for several days. Healing takes time.

A root canal–treated tooth could last your lifetime. To ensure the expected 90 to 95 percent success rate, your tooth should be properly restored by your general dentist after the root canal therapy is complete, and it should be checked by a dentist every year.

A dental checkup, or recall, is a visual exam that includes a check on the final restoration and a check on the health of the tissue around the tooth. The dentist is looking for any tenderness of the tooth or its supporting tissues. In addition, he is looking for draining areas from the tissues which would indicate that the infection is not resolving. Finally, no recall exam is complete without an X-ray evaluation. Comparing the X ray taken before treatment with that taken at the recall exam gives the dentist an indication if healing is taking place.

ENDODONTIC SURGERY

The success rate for traditional root canal therapy is very high (90 to 95 percent). Unfortunately, not unlike any other medical procedure, there are always a few that need further treatment. Studies show the success rate for the 5 to 10 percent of root canal treated teeth that need surgical procedures performed is 50 percent at the end of 10 years.

Sometimes a surgical procedure becomes the only realistic treatment option to resolve a problem. For example, a post (a small metal rod cemented into the canal of the tooth to give the tooth extra length) or an irretrievable metal or plastic obstruction (associated with alternative filling methods for root canals) may be blocking the access down the canal of the tooth. There are times when the infection at the apex (end) of the tooth just will not resolve with antibiotics. In these cases, the only way to get rid of the infection is to remove it by performing a surgical procedure. Patients must also remember there is always the risk that when a dentist tries to renegotiate a canal that has had root canal therapy he may perforate (create a hole in) the side of the root. These are only a few of the reasons why endodontic surgery may be necessary. You should talk over the options with your dentist. Get a second opinion if there is any doubt in your mind that surgery is not the best, or only, course of action in your particular case. Because they are complicated, surgical procedures are almost always done by a specialist.

Apicoectomies, Apical Curettage, and Retrofillings

The most common endodontic surgical procedures are called *apicoectomies, apical curettage,* and *retrofillings*. These three procedures may be done separately, but they are usually done during the same operation. The treatment depends on the circumstances of the case.

Let us see what happens during endodontic surgery. First, the tooth is anesthetized. Anesthetics with a vasoconstrictor (epinephrine) are preferable because they keep the bleeding to a minimum during surgery. However, if you have a heart condition, it may not be possible to use epinephrine. Check with your dentist.

Second, an incision is made that extends to, at least, one tooth on either side of the tooth needing endodontic surgery. The incision allows the gingival tissue to be retracted (pulled back) to expose the area of the root tip (apex) of the tooth. The root tip is the site of the operation.

Third, the bone over the root tip is removed using a dental drill. This fully exposes the root tip. Often the infection has already made a hole through the bone, thus minimizing the amount of additional bone that must be removed before the dentist has ample access to the root tip area.

At this point, if it has not been settled in advance, the decision is made whether to do an apical curettage (cleaning out the area of infection in the bone above the root apex with a small spoon-shaped surgical instrument) and/or an apicoectomy (removing of the apex of the tooth) and a retrofilling (placing a silver filling in the canal to seal it after the apicoectomy is done). An apicoectomy involves not only doing an apical curettage but also cutting off the root apex (root tip) using a dental drill. This is done because studies have shown that there is a high probability of tiny extra canals that come out the side of the root in this area. This could be the reason that the root canal therapy is failing. Because it is impossible to clean out, much less adequately fill these tiny extra canals, the dentist must surgically remove them to assist healing. In performing this procedure the dentist assumes that all the remaining major root canals are well filled and extend to the proper length, just short of the root canal apex. If so, there should be a good seal between the walls of the root canals and the filling material.

If the above two conditions are met, an apicoectomy will suffice to bring about proper healing. The dentist will then do a heat seal or a cold seal of the filling material, provided the filling material is gutta-percha. This means he will adapt the filling material to the root canal with either a hot or cold instrument. Either sealing technique is to help ensure that the filling material seals the root canal well.

An X-ray film at the recall appointment can aid the dentist in determining if there is continuing bone destruction at the root apex. This helps him determine if the bone is healing. But since there is no way to know if the canal is sealed well, I feel that whenever there is adequate operating space in the site, a retrofilling should be done in conjunction with an apicoectomy. This is the only way the dentist can be sure that the root canal filling is sealing the canal well.

A retrofilling is simply an extension of the apicoectomy. The dentist uses a small drill or ultrasonic instrument tip to place a hole into the center of the cut root tip. This hole is then filled with amalgam (a silver filling). Prior to placing an amalgam the dentist may use a liquid bonding agent to adhere the amalgam to the tooth. It is the amalgam that provides the seal for the root canal. The amalgam is the retrofilling.

The incision site is *sutured* (stitched) back together after the endodontic surgical procedure(s) have been completed. These sutures are usually removed by your dentist after about five to seven days (unless they are sutures that dissolve over a short period of time).

There are many instances when your total tooth cannot be saved. *Bicuspidization, hemisection,* and *root amputation* are three surgical procedures that can be used to save part of a "total" tooth. All three procedures imply that the tooth to be saved has more than one root. In other words, only teeth with two or more roots can undergo bicuspidization, hemisection, or root amputation. In each of these three instances, root canal therapy must be completed on the remaining roots. Otherwise, the remaining roots will abscess. Teeth needing this type of treatment may or may not have had previous root canals done.

Several instances can occur that necessitate the removal of a root of a tooth. These include: a root that has no bone support, a root that has *resorbed* (dissolved) away, a tooth that has a fracture that extends between the two roots of a two-rooted tooth, or a tooth that has a root canal in a root that cannot be cleaned and filled (for whatever reason) and is not amenable to endodontic surgery.

Now let us discuss how each of these three surgical procedures differ and when they are indicated.

Bicuspidization

Bicuspidization, as the name suggests, is the division of a molar into two bicuspids. This procedure is usually done on lower molars. Even though lower molars usually have two roots, they may have three or more canals. Lower molar bicuspidization can only occur when both of the roots are salvagable. This most frequently occurs when the gingiva and bone around the tooth have receded, exposing the *furcation* (the area between the two roots). Prior to treatment, this area acts as a food trap, adding to the gingival and bony irritation. This results in loss of the *periodontium* (the supportive tissues of the tooth). One method of treating this situation is to do root canal therapy on all the canals in the tooth. Then, the molar is divided into two bicuspids by cutting the tooth with the dentist's handpiece (drill). The two teeth just created from the molar are then contoured to eliminate their potential for catching food and bacteria.

Another common reason for doing a bicuspidization is to salvage a tooth that has a fracture that has split the tooth into two bicuspids through a "natural" course of events. One of the segments may even be loose. After root canal therapy on both roots, the tooth is properly cut and contoured into two segments to simulate two adjacent bicuspids. Both segments are prepared to receive two separate crowns. The two crowns may be soldered (or splinted) together for greater stability; however, the crowns must have an area between the segments that can be kept clean by dental floss, etc.

Hemisection

A hemisection entails not only the removal of one or more roots of a multi-rooted tooth but also the removal of part of the crown of the tooth, after root canal therapy has been completed. In bicuspidization, the crowns remain intact. A hemisection is done more frequently when there is periodontal destruction of one or more roots of a tooth. The root is removed because without adequate bone support around the root of the tooth, the other roots of the tooth are potentially jeopardized.

A hemisection can also be done when a fracture is found in a multi-rooted tooth, and it is obvious that only the root and crown of that part of the tooth which is loose must be removed. This saves the portion of the tooth that is solidly anchored in the periodontium (supporting tissues of the tooth).

The chewing surface (occlusal or biting surface) of the tooth is usually reduced in size after a hemisection because with part of the crown removed the tooth now has less root support to withstand chewing forces. Thus, the final restoration is usually narrower and gives less chewing surface.

Root Amputation

Finally, root amputation is just what the term implies; a root of a multi-rooted tooth is amputated after root canal therapy. This is usually done because one (or more) of the roots has lost too much bony support. This loss of bone support, if not treated, can jeopardize the supporting tissues of adjacent tooth roots. The solution is simple. Remove the root that has inadequate root support. Root amputation differs from a hemisection because root amputation saves the crown portion of the tooth. When a hemisection is done only part of the crown of the tooth is left intact, as described above.

Some teeth may require a combination of treatments. For instance, both a hemisection and a bicuspidization may be necessary on the same tooth. Let us take one of the upper three-rooted molars as an example. This tooth may have a fracture that extends through the crown and between two roots. A bicuspidization is done. Yet, this same tooth may have inadequate bone support on one of the other three roots. This root is removed in a hemisection operation. Root canal therapy is necessary on the remaining roots because the pulp is exposed when the roots are amputated or a bicuspidization is done.

POSTOPERATIVE CARE

Let us assume that the surgery has just been done. Here are some steps to follow to maximize healing and not harm the surgical site.

1. Place an ice pack over the outside area of the face, intermittently for about two hours after the operation. The ice pack should be placed on the face for 15 minutes and then taken off for 15 minutes. This will help to minimize the swelling and bruising that sometimes accompanies these operations.
2. Do not raise the lip to inspect the operated area. This might tear out some of the sutures (stitches) and hamper proper healing.
3. Eat only soft foods for the first 24 hours and be careful not to bite your lip and/or cheeks. Many dentists feel you should avoid carbonated or alcoholic beverages. The tooth and tissues will be sore anyway, so this is an easy order with which to comply. Some anesthetics last a prolonged time. Eating "normal" foods could tear out the sutures, and you could literally chew up a numb lip or cheek.
4. Do not brush the teeth near the operated area. It is best to use a Q-Tip with toothpaste on it to clean the affected teeth. Some dentists recommend placing chlorhexidine on a small piece of gauze and wiping the affected area. Do this gently! By all means, brush the teeth in the rest of the mouth to keep the number of oral microorganisms to a minimum.
5. Use warm saltwater containing one-half of a teaspoon of salt to an 8 ounce glass of warm water, starting the day *after* the surgery. Rinse

and soak the operated site after each meal and before bedtime. This will not only help keep the area clean of food debris but also stimulate a healthy circulation of blood in the tissues to promote healing in the operated site.

6. Get plenty of rest and be sure to take in adequate food, especially liquids such as fruit juices, soups, and milk. This is good advice for any healing process.

7. Take all medications as prescribed. Some studies have shown that 80 percent of all patients do not take their prescribed drugs correctly. Antibiotics are especially important to take properly. They were given for a reason: to get rid of infection.

The only "minor surgery" is a surgery that is done on someone else! There are risks with any operation. The main problems with endodontic surgery are facial swelling and/or bruising. This usually disappears within a week.

A risk of surgery includes *parasthesia* (paralysis) when a lower molar is surgerized. Parasthesia can be temporary or sometimes even permanent. It is caused by nerve damage that occurs during manipulation of the tissue. When surgery is done in the upper teeth, you run a risk of infection that could spread to the sinuses. Infection in the lower teeth can spread to the neck area. There, again, is good reason to take your antibiotics faithfully.

Should any problems with pain, bleeding, etc. occur, do not hesitate to call your dentist at any time. He cannot help you if he does not know you have a problem.

In summary, almost any tooth may be saved if you are willing to go to the trouble and the expense. The above options for teeth that have combined periodontal and endodontic problems have been documented to be reasonably successful. If you really want to save a tooth, talk over these options with your dentist. Usually he will refer you to a specialist for treatment if these more complicated procedures are necessary.

RETREATMENT OF ROOT CANAL THERAPY

The success rate for root canal therapy on a tooth that has never had root canal treatment before is 90 to 95 percent. Thus, between 5 and 10 percent of the teeth that have undergone traditional root canal therapy fail to heal or the pain persists in spite of the treatment. There are also times when a tooth that has responded to traditional root canal therapy becomes painful or diseased months or even years later. When this occurs the tooth can often be saved if a second endodontic procedure is performed. This procedure, called a *retreatment*, involves reopening the tooth so the canals can be cleaned, shaped, filled, and sealed again.

Research studies show that retreatment cases have an 85 percent success rate at the end of 10 years. When a tooth is first diagnosed as needing root canal therapy the pulp (the soft inner tissue of the tooth) is damaged or diseased. Although the pulp is removed during root canal therapy and replaced with a filling material, the tooth is still alive and drawing nourishment from the surrounding gums and bone. Sometimes this living tooth experiences new problems that make it necessary for it to be retreated.

There are several reasons that make retreatment necessary. A common problem that occurs is many times the canals are so small, curved, or filled with tissue that has calcified (hardened) that the tiny instruments used to clean and shape them cannot completely pass through. There are also times when the canals are so small that it is impossible to find, clean, and shape them. If new decay is allowed to remain untreated or if a filling is loose, cracked, or broken it can expose the root canal filling material to bacteria in the saliva that causes new infection in the tooth, making retreatment necessary. Trauma on the tooth can cause it to fracture or to develop a cystic infection around the root tip. In my own practice I have noticed that many times patients who have procrastinated about getting a crown placed on a posterior (back) tooth eventually return to my office needing a retreatment.

Even though all dentists receive some endodontic training in dental school, retreatments are usually performed by an endodontist. They have advanced training in performing complicated procedures such as retreatments, which are more difficult than the original treatment.

Alternatives to retreatment are surgery (already discussed) or extraction. However, since you have already made an investment in saving your tooth, it makes sense to have the tooth retreated to save your investment. If you have the tooth removed, it is necessary to have a replacement tooth in the space so the adjoining teeth in your mouth will not shift, causing you difficulty in biting or chewing. Teeth that are allowed to shift also lead to the development of gum disease or the loss of additional teeth. Replacement teeth can be implanted or attached to healthy teeth via a bridge, but these are expensive procedures. When it comes to efficient chewing and biting there is no substitute for your own tooth.

It is customary for the patient to be charged a fee for a retreatment because an entirely new procedure has to be performed. Most insurance companies allow coverage for retreatments. Check with your employer or insurance company before treatment is started to be sure.

CRACKED TOOTH SYNDROME

Cracked tooth syndrome (CTS) is an incomplete fracture of the dental structures (the tooth). It is practically impossible to detect a cracked tooth on an X ray. Sometimes if the crack occurs in the coronal portion of the tooth it can be detected by shining a special high-intensity light (fiber optic) on the suspected tooth to expose the crack. CTS is usually characterized by sharp pain when the patient bites his teeth together, or more commonly, on the release of the bite. Asking a patient to bite on a wet cotton roll that is placed between the affected teeth is an excellent diagnostic aid for CTS. The pain occurs because tooth structures move or allow fluid to penetrate the crack resulting in pain originating from the pulp or the attachment tissue. The patient also many times develops a sensitivity to cold.

It is generally accepted that the prognosis is poor for saving a tooth with CTS if it has any of the following:

1. a periodontal pocket formation
2. a crack that runs across the floor of the pulp chamber
3. visible mobility of the segments of the tooth

Usually the dentist must rely on symptoms described by the patient and elimination of all other possible causes of the pain before he makes a diagnosis of CTS.

If the dentist feels the prognosis is good for saving a tooth with CTS, it is always necessary to place a crown on the tooth. Many times the tooth is prepared for a final crown and a temporary crown is then placed on the tooth for six weeks to three months to see if the symptoms subside. If symptoms persist, it is necessary for the tooth to have root canal therapy. If the tooth becomes asymptomatic, the final crown is usually cemented on the tooth.

With improvements in dentin bonding agents, it is now possible to internally bond the coronal portion of the tooth together. When the tooth is bonded together it reduces the movement of the tooth structures, thus reducing or eliminating pain when the patient bites together or releases. If the tooth remains asymptomatic it should be restored with a final crown. Internal bonding must be viewed as an experimental approach; as such, the results are not totally predictable.

RESTORING ENDODONTICALLY TREATED TEETH

All teeth that have had endodontic treatment need a timely final restoration to ensure a favorable prognosis. For years there was little scientific rationale available concerning restorative techniques for endodontically treated teeth. Many textbooks directed dentists to restore all endodontically treated teeth with a *post and core buildup* (a metal post surrounded with a filling material that is placed in the upper two-thirds of a root canal–treated tooth to provide length for the tooth and support for the final crown) before the final crown was placed. Dentists believed all endodontically treated teeth were brittle and required extensive restoration. Furthermore, when a lesion was present on the X ray, dentists were taught to wait months for the lesion to heal before the final restoration was placed on the tooth. Recent scientific evidence and technological advances have provided dentists with new perspectives on these and other restorative issues.

Authorities now feel that all endodontically treated teeth need to be restored in a timely manner. Exposing an endodontically treated tooth to saliva compromises the seal and could lead to a need for retreatment. In addition, the unrestored endodontically treated tooth is susceptible to fracture, which could lead to loss of the tooth. Since modern endodontic treatment has such a high success rate, postponing the final restoration for an extended period of time is unnecessary and places the tooth at risk. If the final restoration cannot be placed within a few weeks of the endodontic treatment, a strong, leak-resistant, protective temporary restoration is indicated.

Several factors need to be considered when choosing a final restoration. Critical considerations include the amount of remaining sound tooth structure, the opposing teeth that remain, the position of the tooth in the dental arch, and the length, width, and curvature of the roots of the endodontically treated tooth. It is important to understand that after teeth are treated endodontically they are weaker and may be more likely to break. Since the amount of tooth structure remaining directly affects the strength of the tooth, the strongest teeth are those with the most sound tooth structure remaining.

In anterior (front) teeth with most of the tooth structure remaining the treatment of choice is a dentin-bonded composite resin. If the tooth is discolored it should be bleached before a veneer or crown is placed to insure the best esthetics without needing to remove sound tooth structure. Teeth that lack adequately sound tooth structure may require a post and core buildup before a full-coverage crown is placed.

Since posterior (back) teeth opposing natural teeth must withstand the forces of biting, most contemporary authorities recommend the placement of a protective restoration with full coverage of the cusps of the tooth (e.g. a crown or an onlay).

It is very important to understand that the primary purpose of a post is to retain a core that can be used to support the final restoration. *Posts are for length, not strength.* Posts do not reinforce endodontically treated teeth, and a post is not necessary when there is substantial tooth structure present after a tooth has been prepared. In fact, placing a post can cause a tooth to be more likely to fracture. Posts should not exceed more than one-third of the root diameter. The amount of tooth structure that has to be removed to accommodate a larger post weakens the tooth.

If a tooth has broken off at or below the gum line it is sometimes necessary to do a procedure called *crown lengthening* in order to make the tooth erupt so there will be more tooth structure available for the post and core buildup and crown. This procedure has traditionally been accomplished by removing some tissue to expose some of the root of the tooth to give access to more tooth structure for support of the crown. New technology has now enabled this procedure to be accomplished by attaching *"space age" wires* made of a super-elastic material (nickel-titanium) that exert steady, gentle pressure on the tooth, causing it to erupt. The wires are removed as soon as the tooth has been adequately extruded.

Most authorities agree that it is not acceptable to retreat teeth with paste fills or silver points (cones) before a post is placed. Endodontists I have spoken with agree that the rubberlike substance gutta-percha is the filling material of choice for placement in endodontically treated teeth.

INFORMED CONSENT—
YOUR RIGHT TO ASK

As a general rule, informed consent is satisfied after the dentist who will perform the treatment has discussed in language understood by the patient all relevant information related to the proposed procedure, so as to assist the patient in making an informed decision with respect to undergoing the proposed treatment. Keep in mind that there is always an alternative to every treatment or procedure. There is always the alternative of no treatment at all, and the results of this choice should also be explained.

The American Dental Association (ADA) recommends that dentists have an "informed consent" statement for patients to sign and date (legal guardian if under 18 years old). Most informed consent statements concerning root canal therapy are similar to this: "I understand that root canal treatment is a procedure to retain a tooth which may otherwise require extraction. Although root canal therapy has a very high degree of clinical success, it is still a biological procedure, so it cannot be guaranteed. Occasionally, a tooth which has had root canal therapy may require retreatment, surgery, or even extraction."

Endodontists usually add the following statement: "I also understand that only the root canal treatment is to be performed at this office. The final (outside or 'permanent') restoration (filling, onlay, crown, etc.) will be done by my regular dentist." The written consent form cannot be used as a substitute for the doctor's discussion with each individual patient.

The dentist cannot foresee every possible complication nor convey years of knowledge learned in dental school or in patient care in a few minutes' conversation with you. But there are basic questions that you have the right to ask *before* you are treated. These include:

1. Do you think the tooth should be saved? Why?
2. Do you think that the tooth can be restored? If so, what are the ideal ways to restore it?
3. What do you estimate the cost of the root canal and the restoration to be?
4. Do you use a rubber dam to isolate the tooth being treated? If not, how do you protect me and the tooth?
5. What type of filling material do you use to fill the root canal? Do you use a sealer? Are these materials commonly used by endodontists? If not, why do you use them?
6. Will I have a temporary filling when you are through today? If more than one appointment is needed, how many times do you anticipate that I will need to come back?
7. What problems do you anticipate in the treatment?
8. What are my chances of needing some type of surgery to save this tooth? Will surgery be necessary in the future?
9. When should I go ahead and have a final filling placed?
10. How often should this tooth have a follow-up exam?
11. Do I need antibiotics and/or pain medications?

Informed consent applies to all areas of dentistry. Questions, such as in the example above, should be asked by the patient before any treatment is started. The American Dental Association has encouraged all dentists to discuss with patients in language they can understand any problems they have identified that need treatment, and the treatment recommendations. Then the dentist should provide informed consent forms to the patient to read, sign, and date before any treatment is started. This will insure that all patients understand the treatment proposed, alternatives to that proposed treatment, and the consequences of no treatment at all.

Do not be shy! When in doubt, talk it out! It is your right to ask questions. Use this right and be a better consumer.

FOCAL INFECTION THEORY

At this writing, research has demonstrated that the theory of focal infection was wrong. The original research that was widely accepted in the early 1900s, when it was introduced by Dr. Weston Price, is no longer considered by dental authorities to be valid. Dr. Price's research seemed to indicate that oral bacteria could be trapped in your tooth during routine dental treatment, and then either the bacteria or the toxins they produce migrate to other parts of your body. It was believed this would lead to cancer, diseases of the kidney, heart, nervous, gastrointestinal, endocrine and other systems, arthritis, and hundreds of other ailments. As a result the theory caused patients to needlessly have endodontically treated teeth extracted. The theory also caused millions of tonsillectomies to be performed, since they were also considered to be a localized area of focal infection.

The introduction of extensive research, both biologically and scientifically based, in the last 50 years has proven beyond a shadow of a doubt the theory of focal infection was wrong. Root canal–treated teeth cannot harm you because when this procedure is performed the soft inner tissue of the tooth that is diseased or damaged is removed, and any bacteria present are destroyed by cleaning and filling the canal space. When endodontic therapy is appropriately performed clinical symptoms should disappear, and radiographic and histologic healing of the area at the apex of the tooth should occur. Millions and millions of root canal treatments are successfully performed on teeth each year throughout the world. Most health care practitioners are in agreement that accepted root canal procedures are safe, effective, and help you keep your natural teeth for a lifetime.

4

Oral Pathology

Oral pathology is a specialty concerned with the diagnosis of oral diseases, including cancer. A recognized oral pathologist must complete a two- to three-year, ADA-approved training program beyond dental school. Oral pathologists most often work at dental schools or research labs/clinics. The *direct* need of a patient for specialists in this area of expertise would be rare. Their purpose is more for consultation with either your general dentist or your dental specialist.

The *indirect* need for the services of an oral pathologist is very important in treating a range of problems. The type of problem for which an oral pathologist might be called in is tissue identification (soft or bony) that is beyond the range of normal.

Most authorities agree that a tissue specimen from the area of the root apex should be sent to an oral pathologist if there is any suspicion of a problem beyond what endodontic surgery can resolve. The oral pathologist can inform the dentist if there is some bodily malfunction that has caused the bone loss. Over 30 reasons exist for continuing bone destruction, including some very exotic diseases, tumors, cysts, or cancer that has migrated via the bloodstream into the jaws. For example, in a recently reported case, Hodgkin's disease was determined as the cause of a patient's jaw bone loss. The oral pathologist can also identify *erythroplakia*, a known precancerous problem that may show up as a red area in the mouth, and *leukoplakia*, another precancerous condition commonly seen inside the cheeks of 50–70-year-old men that is signaled by a white area in the mouth. White patches could also be the first sign of AIDS. Authorities recommend that any lump or lesion that has not healed within two weeks of the removal of the cause should be biopsied. The main tools of the oral pathologist are his knowledge, experience, and his microscope. He can make thin specimens that are stained with specific dyes, examine the specimens to determine the types of cells that are present; and from this diagnosis he can determine what treatment the patient needs to resolve the problem. Here is where oral pathologists work closely with other dental specialists and general dentists.

ORAL CANCER

The oral pathologist, besides being involved with pulpal and periapical pathology, is very much involved with the detection of oral cancer. Oral cancer is the sixth most common cancer in the world. Studies show oral cancers are more common than leukemia, melanomia, and cancers of the brain, liver, kidney, stomach, thyroid, ovary, or cervix. Each year in the United States oral cancer strikes 43,000 people, with a five-year survival rate of 54 percent, lower for African Americans. Of those diagnosed, 90 percent occur in the over 40-years-of-age group, and males are affected more frequently than females. Statistics further show 95 percent of all oral cancer is squamous cell carcinoma, which is related to tobacco use. Part of the reason oral cancer has such a poor prognosis is that more than half of the cancers have metastasized at the time of diagnosis. Detecting oral cancer early is the key. As an example, one type of oral cancer, when treated while the cancer is still less than a half inch in diameter, has a survival rate of about 60 percent. The same cancer, if not treated until it is double that size, reduces the patient's survival rate to only 15 percent on the average. When diagnosed, surgery is usually required with follow-up radiation and chemotherapy treatments. Many times the surgery is disfiguring, and the radiation and chemotherapy therapy can cause severe complications.

Major risk factors for oral cancer include the use of tobacco products (smoking and chewing), the use of alcohol, exposure to the sun (lip cancer), dietary factors, and exposure to carcinogens in the workplace. All parts of the oral cavity are affected by oral cancer: tongue, lips, floor of the mouth, soft palate, tonsils, back of the throat, and salivary glands. Oral cancers most frequently occur on the lips (usually on the lower lip). This is probably from chronic exposure to the sun, and is especially prevalent in people with a light complexion. The tongue is the second most frequently affected site. These cancers occur most often on the sides and on the back two-thirds of the tongue. The floor of the mouth is the third most frequent site. Cancers of the floor of the mouth and the tongue are the most aggressive and result in the highest death rates, because cancers here spread most frequently to the lymph nodes and then to other parts of the body. The gingiva, roof of the mouth, and the inside of the cheeks are less frequently affected. But oral cancers certainly can and do occur there.

It is estimated that 75 percent of all oral and pharyngeal cancers are caused by excessive smoking and heavy consumption of alcohol. It is felt by most authorities that alcohol promotes the effects of carcinogens found in tobacco.

Smokeless tobacco is a dangerous substance that has been proven to cause oral cancer. In addition, it has also been proven in numerous studies to cause periodontal disease, tooth loss, leukoplakias, and risk of heart attacks, high blood pressure, strokes, and kidney diseases. A campaign is now under way by several health organizations to educate the public about the hazards of smokeless tobacco. Athletes are being encouraged to tell young people not to use this product in order to discourage its use. Many young people who use smokeless tobacco have already experienced lesions, but almost none have talked to an adult or health personnel about the problem.

The American Dental Association has just recently introduced an insurance code (01320) to be used by dentists to cover charges for tobacco intervention treatment. Dental consumers need to be cognizant of this new dental benefit code so plan purchasers and third-party payers can be encouraged to include it in their dental benefit contracts. Dentists are also being encouraged to prescribe nicotine patches to smokers to help them overcome their addiction.

A recent CDC study revealed that only 14.3 percent of Americans have had an oral cancer screening. By the year 2000 the U.S. Public Health Service's Oral Health 2000 objective is that at least 40 percent of the over-50 Americans will be screened at least once a year for oral cancer. This would allow the disease to be caught earlier when it is localized and more treatable. Dental health professionals have the greatest opportunity to identify oral cancer while it is asymptomatic, innocuous, and unsuspected. They usually see patients twice a year, and the exam can easily be incorporated into this checkup. It only takes about two minutes to do an oral cancer exam. According to the National Cancer Institute and the National Institute of Dental Research, a three-part examination of the mouth includes the extraoral head and neck areas, the intraoral soft tissue, and the dental and periodontal tissues. When examining inside the mouth the dentist usually wraps gauze around the tongue and pulls it forward. He then feels and looks at the tissue under the tongue and inside the cheeks for texture or color changes, bleeding, lesions, masses, ulcerations, lymphadenopathy (swollen lympth nodes).

The FDA is currently reviewing a new diagnostic system called OraScan that is being developed by Zila Pharmaceuticals (Phoenix,

Arizona). This system incorporates a series of oral rinse solutions to enhance the visualization of abnormal tissue. The disclosing agent leaves areas of unhealthy cells clearly defined in blue, allowing the disease to be diagnosed in its early, more treatable stages. A dentist can complete the OraScan diagnostic procedure in less than five minutes as an adjunct to a routine checkup.

Warning: Do not wait for pain to tell you that something is wrong. If a mouth sore does not heal in two weeks, seek the opinion of your dentist. Early diagnosis can save your life.

Look for these other warning signs:

1. a sore on the lips, gingiva, or inside the mouth that bleeds easily and does not heal within two weeks
2. a lump or thickening in the cheek that can be felt with the tongue.
3. a numbness or loss of feeling in any part of your mouth
4. soreness in the mouth or a feeling that something is caught in the throat with no known cause
5. a white or red patch on the gums, tongue, inside of the mouth
6. difficulty in chewing or swallowing food

The value of self-examination is strictly for screening purposes. When questions arise, your dentist is the best source of information about any suspicious sores in and around the mouth and neck areas. Make sure an examination for oral cancer is included in your check-up when you see your dentist. If your dentist feels you have a suspicious lesion he will probably do a biopsy. This involves taking a tissue specimen from the affected area and sending it to pathologist so he can examine it under a microscope to determine the cells present in the area.

Thus, the oral pathologist is primarily a resource person for the general dentists and specialists. His scope of concern ranges from identifying the causes of dental caries, to periodontal disease, to oral signs of exotic diseases, to the detection and cure of oral cancers.

ANTIBIOTIC THERAPY FOR DENTAL PROCEDURES

Infective Endocarditis

Infective endocarditis (IE) is a serious heart infection that can occur when microorganisms enter the bloodstream and work their way to the heart. This is risky for patients with heart abnormalities because the bacteria may cause bacterial endocarditis (a serious inflammation of the heart valves or tissues). Symptoms of IE do not occur until from a few days to a few weeks after the microorganisms enter the bloodstream. This makes it difficult to determine exactly what incident was responsible for the infection. However, if no dental treatment has occurred within four weeks of the onset of the symptoms, the dental procedure can probably be ruled out as the cause of IE.

Numerous studies have confirmed that when the recommended regimen of antibiotics is taken the incidence of bacteria is reduced. Since gingival bleeding can occur with most dental procedures the American Heart Association (AHA) recommends antibiotic prophylaxis with all dental procedures, including professional tooth cleaning for high risk cardiac patients.

The newest recommendation by the American Heart Association is the use of chlorhexidine or similar agents before tooth extraction. It is recommended that chlorhexidine be used to irrigate the area where the extraction will occur. Then chlorhexidine should be painted on isolated and dried gingiva in the area three to five minutes before the extraction is accomplished. This will reduce postextraction bacteremia. The use of chlorhexidine should be used as an adjunct (not a substitute) to recommended antibiotic prophylaxis, particularly in high-risk patients and/or with poor oral hygiene.

Recent studies indicate dental procedures cause about 4 percent of all IE cases. The American Heart Association and the Council on Scientific Affairs of the American Dental Association have jointly recommended the following antibiotic prophylaxis (see table) for the prevention of IE in high risk patients who have:

- a prosthetic heart valve (bioprosthetic or homograft)
- a history of endocarditis (even if no history of heart disease has been diagnosed)
- most congenital cardiac malformations
- an organic heart murmur
- hypertrophic cardiomyopathy
- a mitral valve prolapse with valvular regurgitation
- a surgically constructed systemic pulmonary shunt
- rheumatic or other acquired valvular dysfunction, even after valve surgery

Patients who have been diagnosed with the following are considered low risk and do not need to be premedicated prophylactically:

- heart murmurs that are functional, physiological, or innocent

FOR DENTAL/ORAL/UPPER RESPIRATORY TRACT PROCEDURES

I. Standard Regimen in Patients at Risk (includes those with prosthetic heart valves and other high-risk patients):

Amoxicillin 3.0 g orally one hour before procedure, then 1.5 g six hours after initial dose.★

For amoxicillin/penicillin-allergic patients:

Erythromycin ethylsuccinate 800 mg or erythromycin stearate 1.0 g orally two hours before a procedure, then one-half the dose six hours after the initial administration.★

or

Clindamycin 300 mg orally one hour before a procedure and 150 mg six hours after initial dose.★

II. Alternate Prophylactic Regimens for Dental/Oral/Upper Respiratory Tract Procedures in Patients at Risk:

A. For patients unable to take oral medications:

Ampicillin 2.0 g IV (or IM) 30 minutes before procedure, then ampicillin 1.0 g IV (or IM) *or* amoxicillin 1.5 g orally six hours after initial dose.★

or

For ampicillin/amoxicillin/penicillin-allergic patients unable to take oral medications:

Clindamycin 300 mg IV 30 minutes before a procedure and 150 mg IV (or orally) six hours after initial dose.★

B. For patients considered to be at high risk who are not candidates for the standard regimen:

Ampicillin 2.0 g IV (or IM) plus gentamicin 1.5 mg/kg IV (or IM) (not to exceed 80 mg) 30 minutes before procedure, followed by amoxicillin 1.5 g orally six hours after the initial dose. Alternatively, the parenteral regimen may be repeated eight hours after the initial dose.★

For amoxicillin/ampicillin/penicillin-allergic patients considered to be at high risk:

Vancomycin 1.0 g IV administered over one hour, starting one hour before the procedure. No repeat dose is necessary.★

◆ a history of rheumatic fever without heart murmur
◆ mitral valve prolapse without regurgitation
◆ cardiac pacemakers and implanted defibrillators
◆ surgical repair without residual beyond six months of
    secundum artrial septal defects
    ventricular septal defects
    patent ductus arteriosus
◆ previous coronary graft surgery.

*Note: Initial pediatric dosages are listed below. Follow-up oral dose should be one-half the initial dose. Total pediatric dose should not exceed total adult dose.

Amoxicillin:†	50 mg/kg	Vancomycin:	20 mg/kg
Clindamycin:	10 mg/kg	Ampicillin:	50 mg/kg
Erythromycin ethyl succinate or stearate:	20 mg/kg	Gentamicin:	2.0 mg/kg

†The following weight ranges may also be used for the initial pediatric dose of amoxicillin:

<15 kg (33 lbs), 750 mg

15–30 kg (33–66 lbs), 1500 mg

>30 kg (66 lbs), 3000 mg (full adult dose)

Kilogram to pound conversion chart: (1 kg = 2.2 lb)

kg	lb
5	11.0
10	22.0
20	44.0
30	66.0
40	88.0
50	110.0

Adapted from *Prevention of Bacterial Endocarditis: Recommendations by the American Heart Association* by the Committee on Rheumatic Fever, Endocarditis, and Kawasaki Disease.

JAMA 1990; 264: 2919–2922, © 1990 American Medical Association (also excerpted in *J Am Dent Assoc* 1991; 122: 87–92).

Please refer to these joint American Heart Association–American Dental Association recommendations for more complete information as to which patients and which procedures require prophylaxis.

◆ previous Kawasaki disease without valvular dysfunction
◆ Isolated secundum atrial septal defect

The new recommendations of amoxicillin as the first-choice antibiotic for dental procedures replaces the 1984 AHA recommendations for penicillin V, especially if the patient is high risk and is being offered oral antibiotics. The use of tetracyclines and sulfonamides are not recommended for endocarditis prophylaxis.

Patients who are already taking antibiotics (or have taken them within the last week) will have high levels of resistant strains of bacteria. Therefore, the American Heart Association (AHA) recommends that one of the alternative antibiotics be given in addition. For example, if a patient is already taking penicillin then he has high levels of resistence to penicillin/amoxicillin organisms. Therefore, he should take erythromycin or clindamycin in addition. An alternative would be to wait one week after completing the penicillin before having the dental procedure accomplished so he could safely take amoxicillin.

Poor oral hygiene and periodontal (gum) disease can spread bacteria that threaten the heart even in the absence of dental procedures. Good oral hygiene, not antibiotic prophylaxis for dental procedures, is universally accepted as the best preventive for infective endocarditis originating in the oral cavity. It is very important to establish and maintain good oral health by brushing, flossing, and using a mouth rinse each day. Be sure to see your dentist regularly.

Prosthetic Joints

Both the American Dental Association and the American Academy of Oral Medicine feel that due to a lack of scientific information they do not recommend routine antibiotic prophylaxis for patients with prosthetic joints. They do, however, recommend that dentists consult with the patient's orthopedic surgeon on an individual basis to determine the need for prophylaxis. When indicated, many physicians recommend a cephalosporin antibiotic regimen. Whenever possible, it is recommended that all active infection should be treated before the surgical placement of a joint prosthesis.

5

Oral and Maxillo-facial Surgery

Your general dentist can handle most types of dental procedures that require minor surgery. However, any surgical procedure, no matter how minor, can lead to complications such as uncontrolled bleeding, pain, or spread of infection. In rare instances, surgical complications can even become life threatening. When a general dentist feels treatment involving surgery needs the expertise of a dental specialist in this area, he refers the patient to an oral and maxillofacial surgeon.

A board-eligible specialist in oral and maxillofacial surgery must complete a three-year, ADA-approved training program beyond dental school. The oral surgeon only performs dental procedures that require some type of surgical intervention, and he is limited to surgical procedures involving the head and neck area. Even though oral surgeons perform most surgical procedures in their offices, they are usually on staff at area hospitals so they can also do more complicated procedures in a hospital setting.

Oral surgeons are also involved in diagnosing and treating injuries and birth defects that affect the mouth, jaws, and neck area. Additionally, they can administer a variety of sedations (to relieve anxiety) and anesthetics that most general dentists, or other types of specialists, are not adequately trained to administer.

A large part of the oral surgeon's practice is extraction of teeth. Not all teeth are treatable, and in fact, it is not even desirable to save all teeth. For example, sometimes there is not enough room for all the teeth in your mouth. In these cases, an orthodontist may be consulted, and an oral surgeon will remove selected teeth to provide adequate room for the remaining teeth. Some teeth, such as impacted third molars (wisdom teeth), often need to be extracted. More about that later in this chapter!

Before any hospital surgery is done on a patient, the oral surgeon must first do a "workup" of both the patient's medical history and present medical condition to insure that the patient can safely undergo the surgical procedure. The age, mental attitude, and the patient's general health must all be taken into consideration. Special precautions are required for those patients with: blood or circulatory disease, heart disease, diabetes, respiratory infections, severe active infections, or those who are pregnant. Elderly and epileptic patients are very likely to incur accidents requiring an oral surgeon. These special precautions usually require the oral surgeon to consult and work closely with the patient's physician.

Fractures and dislocations of bones of the face and/or jaws are often treated by oral and maxillofacial surgeons. In treating such injuries the oral surgeon usually must work in a hospital operating room, where he will wire and splint the bones back into place. One advantage that the oral and maxillofacial surgeon has in treating any of these head and neck injuries is that he is a dentist. This background gives him a greater appreciation of how teeth should relate in proper occlusion (bite), which saves much postoperative treatment as it relates to the patient's ability to chew after healing has occurred.

Oral surgeons are often referred patients who might have cancer. Thus, the oral surgeon performs many biopsies. If the oral pathologist reports that the patient has cancer, the oral surgeon will become a part of a team effort to save the patient's life. Treatment of oral cancer may require extensive surgery and/or X-ray or radiation therapy. Most likely, it is the oral surgeon who removes a portion of the diseased oral tissue, if this becomes necessary. This could entail removal of a part of the jaw, tongue, or roof of the mouth. This all sounds very frightening, but such measures often save lives.

The oral surgeon is also involved with treating babies born with a *cleft lip* (also called a harelip) since it looks like a rabbit's lip which is normally split. This surgical procedure is usually performed soon after birth. The scar usually disappears as the child gets older. Studies show that one baby in a thousand is born with a cleft lip. There is also strong evidence that cleft lips can be hereditary.

A *cleft palate* (also appearing in one birth in a thousand) occurs when there is a direct opening between the roof of the mouth, the palate, and the floor of the nose. When the baby tries to eat, the food will come out of its nose. The treatment necessary to correct this birth defect is much more complex than that for the cleft lip. The cleft palate operation is generally done when the child is one to two years of age. In some cases, several operations are necessary to complete the closure of the palate.

After surgery, the child will need extensive speech therapy and orthodontics. Complete rehabilitation requires a team of specialists that includes an oral surgeon, an orthodontist, a prosthodontist, a general dentist, a speech therapist, a physician, and, on occasion, a psychologist, a psychiatrist, and a hearing specialist.

Technology today enables oral surgeons to use lasers (a beam of light energy) and radiosurgery (high-frequency radio waves) as alternatives or in conjunction with traditional surgical equipment. Both of these methods offer rapid tissue removal with minimal trauma to the tissue and increased visibility because there is a significant decrease in bleeding. Today's technology also offers improved microscopes for better visibility when performing surgical procedures.

WISDOM TEETH . . . IS IT WISE TO KEEP THEM?

Wisdom teeth, which are located behind the second (12-year) molars, generally erupt between 17 and 21 years of age. They can be an asset if they are healthy and properly positioned in the mouth. However, since this is not always the case, patients are sometimes advised to have these teeth removed in order to protect their overall oral health. The American Dental Association recommends extraction when the following occurs:

1. Wisdom teeth only partially erupt. This is a problem because bacteria are able to enter around the tooth and cause an infection (known as *pericoronitis*), which results in pain, swelling, and tenderness in the jaw area. If the infection extends into the bone supporting the roots, it may become even more serious. This condition is called *osteomyelitis*. Bony infections are difficult to treat. Often large doses of antibiotics for long periods of time are recommended.

2. *Impacted* wisdom teeth (teeth not able to fully erupt) continue to try to break through the gum tissue and into alignment in the mouth, even if there is not enough room to accommodate them. The continued pressure caused by the eruption process can eventually destroy the healthy second molar teeth. Many times the roots of the healthy teeth dissolve away, a process called *root resorption*. This can occur with no perceptible symptoms, and thus will only be detected through an X-ray examination of the affected area.

3. A fluid-filled cyst (sac) or tumor forms, destroying the surrounding bone and tooth-root structures.

If a tooth is in proper position, its removal is no more complicated than any other tooth. However, I would recommend an oral and maxillofacial surgeon perform removal of a tooth that is not in proper position and, thus, cannot erupt. This condition is termed a *bony impaction*.

Extractions can be performed with either local or general anesthesia. Many patients want to "go to sleep" (general anesthesia) for this type of procedure. During their specialty education program training oral surgeons are trained in a hospital setting to use general (IV) sedation. For this reason, they usually have the proper equipment and training to be able to safely offer this type of anesthesia in their office.

The ADA recommends that people 16 to 19 years of age have their wisdom teeth evaluated to see if they need to be removed. Teeth removed before age 20 have fewer complications because the roots of the teeth are not yet fully developed, the surrounding bone is softer, and there is less chance of damaging nerves or other structures. Authorities agree most dental-related surgical complications occur in patients who are over 30 years of age. Some patients experience *paresthesia* (a numbness or tingling) in the jaw area following surgery. Normal sensation usually returns in time.

Postoperative Instructions for Tooth Extractions

Tooth extractions are usually minor surgical procedures. It is expected the area will heal in a few days. In the meantime, here are a few guidelines to help promote healing, prevent complications, and help make you more comfortable.

1. After an extraction your dentist will place a gauze pack on the extraction site so that you may apply pressure by biting firmly to limit bleeding while clotting takes place. Leave the pack in place for 30 to 45 minutes after you leave the dental office. If there is still bleeding when it is time to remove the packing, put a new pack in place and maintain pressure for another 30 minutes. Replace the pack, as necessary, with a clean pack, if it becomes soaked with blood or saliva.

2. Never suck on the extraction site. This will disturb the blood clot that needs to form in the tooth socket for normal healing. For the first 24 hours after an extraction it is also recommended that you don't smoke, rinse your mouth vigorously, or clean the teeth next

to the extraction site. You should also drink through a straw and limit strenuous activity. Failure to follow these suggestions could result in delayed healing and/or a *dry socket.*

3. Be careful not to bite your cheek, lip, or tongue while the area is numb. The numbness will subside within a few hours, depending on the type of anesthetic used.

A small amount of blood may leak from the extraction site until a clot forms. However, you should call your dentist if heavy bleeding continues after you get home. Remember, a lot of saliva and a little blood can look like a lot of bleeding.

You may experience some pain and swelling after a tooth is extracted. It usually helps to apply an ice pack to the face for 15 minutes, and then remove for 15 minutes. Repeat this as necessary. If medication is prescribed by your dentist be sure to take it as directed. If it does not seem to work do not increase the dosage without first consulting your dentist. If you have prolonged or severe pain, swelling, bleeding, or fever you should call your dentist so you can be given instructions on how to care for your problem.

Be sure to drink lots of liquids and eat soft, healthful foods after an extraction. *Avoid alcoholic or carbonated beverages and hot liquids.* You should begin eating solid food the next day if you can chew comfortably. It is a good idea to chew on the opposite side of the extraction site for at least two days.

Begin gently rinsing your mouth with warm salt water (one-half teaspoon of salt in an 8 oz. glass of warm water) the day after the extraction. *Do not swallow the salt water.* Rinsing gently after meals keeps food particles out of the extraction site. Do not use a mouth rinse or mouthwash during the early stages of the healing period.

It is important to continue to keep the remainder of your teeth clean and flossed after an extraction. Brushing the tongue will help eliminate the bad breath and unpleasant taste that is associated with an extraction. Use a soft-bristled brush so that the tissues in your mouth are not injured.

ORTHOGNATHIC SURGERY ... WHAT IS IT?

Most people think in terms of orthodontics to change the way their teeth look. But orthodontics is limited to changing the position of teeth to improve their appearance. Orthodontics cannot correct malformations of the bones of the face. This surgery, which is called *orthognathic* surgery, is usually done by an oral and maxillofacial surgeon in the hospital.

The most common problem encountered by patients who need orthognathic surgery is when the patient's upper and lower jaws are not the same size. This is usually a hereditary problem. The surgeon can cut the upper and/or lower jaw and move the segments to a location that allows better functioning of the teeth, while also giving the patient balanced facial esthetics. There are also certain skeletal irregularities that require surgical intervention.

If your child has an obvious problem, he/she should have a consultation appointment with both an orthodontist and an oral and maxillofacial surgeon by the age of six to eight. First, the specialist will determine if a problem exists in the growth and development of the facial structure. Second, if a problem is found, a treatment plan is made for future correction. This allows early intervention to simplify surgical correction. By the time the child is 11 or 12, some problems, such as receding chins and overbites, can be corrected.

This early intervention, it is thought, allows the child to be spared some of the trauma of having a disfigurement during adolescence. The surgery can be a factor in shaping the child's adult appearance, which can have a tremendous impact on his life. Additional benefits of the surgery are the ability to breathe and eat better and to enunciate words more clearly.

Risks and costs are considerations before having cosmetic, surgical intervention to change your facial features. The benefits are often very personal. It is important that you determine whether the surgical risks are worth the benefits. You must keep in mind that quite possibly surgery will not bring about the benefits you desire. Maybe what you really need to change is a poor self-image that neither surgery nor orthodontics can correct. The question that is often most difficult to answer is: Do poor self-images occur independently of facial features, or are they a result of facial features?

The oral surgeon and the orthodontist should work closely to determine how best to correct the problems of patients who need orthognathic surgery. This "team" uses plaster models of the teeth and special X-ray films to make their calculations before beginning treatment. With the new technology of today, many dental professionals are using computer diagnostic and imaging systems to allow both the doctor and the patient a clear understanding of treatment objectives and possible outcomes. The orthodontist frequently corrects the occlusion both before and after the surgery. The cost of this surgery varies, depending on the extent of the problem and the time involved in correcting it.

As with any major surgical procedure, the patient usually is admitted to the hospital the night before the surgery is to take place. The procedure involves making incisions inside the mouth and cheeks to avoid any external scars. In addition, new high-speed saws and drills separate the bones rapidly and at the proper location. The jaws are wired together after the operation to allow the bones to heal in the proper new position. The operation may take several hours to complete. The patient's stay in the hospital can be from a few days to several weeks, depending on the extent of the surgery. The healing time is at least eight to ten weeks. A liquid diet is necessary during the healing period. That makes sense since the teeth are wired together, and the patient cannot chew anyway!

Orthognathic surgery differs from "plastic surgery." Orthognathic surgery involves redesigning the jaws and their immediate surrounding structures. Plastic surgeons usually operate outside the mouth on soft tissues including the ears, eyes, and nose. These latter structures are not in the realm of orthognathic surgery.

Beauty is in the eye of its beholder. The ancient Greeks had a criteria for classic beauty, and many of the oral and maxillofacial surgeons, as well as the plastic surgeons, have adopted a similar criteria for what they consider the "perfect" face. It is as follows: The face should be five times the width of one eye; the face should be symmetrical on both sides of the vertical midline; vertical, parallel lines to the midline of the face should be able to be drawn from the middle of the pupil of the eye to the corner of the mouth; and the distance from the hairline to the bridge of the nose, from the bridge of the nose to the middle of the upper lip, and from the middle of the upper lip to the tip of the chin should all be equal.

Orthognathic surgery is not for everyone. But when indicated, it can make a big difference in how you feel about yourself.

IMPLANTS

Dental implants are metal tooth replacements that are anchored into the bone of the dental ridge. They bring us a step closer to tooth replacements that look natural and feel secure. The evolution of implants has steadily progressed since the late 1950s, when titanium was introduced as a biocompatible metal that would eliminate biological rejection. Titanium has been a significant factor in accelerating the practice of implantology.

Today about 90 percent of general dentists suggest implants to carefully selected patients. Implants should be considered an option when a patient cannot gain comfort in wearing a conventional, removable full or partial denture because of physiological problems (sore spots or a poor ridge) and/or psychological (gag) problems, or as an option to placing a bridge to replace a single tooth because so much healthy tooth structure has to be removed in order to accommodate the crowns. Implants can provide support for one or more teeth so a crown, a fixed bridge, or an overdenture can be placed in the mouth.

Although a single dentist may perform the entire implant process, frequently two or more dentists are involved as a team. Before you are accepted as an implant candidate, your dentist will perform a thorough clinical examination and a complete medical and dental history. Many times the primary dentist will refer the patient to either an oral/maxillo-facial surgeon or a periodontist for surgical placement of the implants. Then the primary dentist makes and fits the replacement teeth.

Implantology is *not* one of the eight ADA dental specialties, and the training and experience of those who perform implants vary. Before you commit yourself to treatment ask the dentist about his education and training with regard to implants, how many implants he has performed, and how long he has been performing them. Dental implants are a complex procedure that require specific knowledge and training. You may even want to get a second opinion. You could also contact a faculty member of your nearest dental school to determine who is best qualified in your area to perform implants.

Implants have three components: the anchor (which may be surgically placed into the bone), a post (which is attached to the anchor), and the artificial tooth (which attaches to the post).

There are several types of implants on the market, but at this time the ADA only considers two to be safe. They are the endosteal and the subperiosteal.

Endosteal implants are placed directly into the jawbone. This implant cannot be used unless the patient has adequate bone support. First, an anchor is placed surgically into the jaw. For best results, the surgeon must do minimal damage to the tissue. Anchors are available in several shapes and are sometimes coated with a material that enables the bone to adhere to it. This process of attachment is called *osteointegration* (the bone integrates or bonds with the implant material). After the anchor(s) is/are submerged it is left undisturbed for three to six months to allow it to firmly adhere to the underlying bone. Then a second surgical procedure is usually needed to connect the post to the anchor. Finally, the artificial tooth (or teeth) is/are attached to the post. This type of implant is often used to secure a fixed bridge.

A *subperiosteal* implant consists of a metal frame that rests upon the jawbone just below the gum tissue, instead of being placed directly into the jawbone. The metal frame is made by using impressions of the surgically exposed jawbone. After the frame is constructed, the gum tissue is reopened and the frame is fitted onto the jawbone. The implant adheres to the jaw as the gum tissue heals. The posts of the implant protrude through the gum. This type of implant is often used to secure an *overdenture* (a tooth replacement for an entire arch that is permanently secured to the implants).

Despite their high success rate some implants are physiologically rejected, must be removed. The primary reasons for failures include peri-implantitis (bony infections), placing the crowns on the anchors prematurely, and insufficient or improper maintenance of the implant site. Other complications include improper alignment, persistent discomfort, and cosmetic problems. Dr. Andrea Mobelli of the University of Bern in Switzerland suggests that patients with a history of periodontal disease may be a greater risk for peri-implantitis because of a higher frequency of periodontal bacteria and increased susceptibility to these organisms.

The ADA states that "dental implants are not for everyone." They stress that all implant candidates must be carefully screened. Candidates must be in good health, have healthy bone and gingiva to support the implant, be psychologically suitable, and be committed to meticulous oral hygiene and regular dental visits. They also must have no current financial difficulties since this procedure is usually more expensive than other methods of tooth replacement. Most insurance companies cover less than 10 percent of the fee for implants. While the procedure usually takes about nine to twelve months to complete, implants can last ten years or longer. Never assume anything is permanent. You will lose your implant if you do not take care of it.

For many years periodontists focused on using *hydroxylapatite* (HA) to rebuild or augment resorbed ridges. Today, periodontology focuses not only on stopping the progression of periodontal disease but also on regenerating lost periodontal supporting structures that previously would have been lost as a result of disease. This has increased the patient's treatment options with regard to implants. Studies have shown a group of commonly used periodontal surgical methods called *guided tissue regeneration* (GTR) are effective in the promotion of tissue healing around implants.

In GTR, a biocompatible membrane is used to isolate the *defect* (area of bone loss) from the gum and connective tissue. The area in question is surgically opened and the membrane is placed very close to the surface of the tooth to prevent the growth of tissue in the defect. This allows the bone and connecting tissue to be able to fill in the space. After about six weeks, the healing is complete and the membrane is removed during a minor surgical procedure. Second-generation GTR is a resorbable membrane that is completely resorbed six to twelve months later. This eliminates the need for a second surgical procedure to remove the membrane. Third-generation GTR systems are still in the research and development stage. They involve adding a bioactive substance (e.g. growth hormone) to the membrane to facilitate growth previously accomplished by the patient's innate healing capacity.

Bone grafting is another form of regeneration. The three classes of bone grafts are *autografts*, *allografts*, and *alloplasts*. Autografts are grafts of the patient's own bone harvested from a separate site on their body (usually the hip area). This provides the most predictable bone fill and periodontal regeneration. Allograft bone is human bone from cadaver donors. Demineralized freeze-dried bone (DFDB) is widely available from regional tissue banks. A disadvantage of this graft is that the amount of growth factors present in DFDB varies based on the donor of the bone. This graft also brings concerns about the transmission of HIV infection in bone. Therefore, it is recommended that clinicians only use DFDB that is obtained from a source that is accredited by the American Association of Tissue Banks, and that uses polymerase chain-reaction DNA testing on allograft bone. The third type of bone graft is alloplast, a synthetic bone substitute. The regenerative potential of synthetic bone grafts has been shown to be very limited.

The results of a bone graft vary with the skill and experience of the clinician and the material used. In addition, the patient's physical condition and compliance with oral hygiene and maintenance affects the outcome. Most authorities agree the autograft with the patient's own bone has the greatest predictability of regeneration with least risk. The best alternative choice is a combination of autograft (grafts of the patient's own bone) and allograft (demineralized freeze-dried bone from an accredited tissue bank). Regeneration techniques permit the placement of implants in sites that previously would not have been possible. GTR has become a routine method of expanding the ridge in the mouth. Implants, in extraction sites, are now more predictable because the ability to maintain bone at these sites has been improved.

6

Orthodontics

O rthodontics is the branch of dentistry concerned with the detection, correction, prevention, and study of irregularities and deformities of the teeth, face, and jaws. The general goals of orthodontic treatment are to establish proper occlusion, improve esthetics, and enhance gingival and periodontal health. The specialist in this field is known as an orthodontist. A recognized orthodontic specialist has received two or more years of education beyond dental school in an ADA-approved orthodontic training program. He is trained to be able to treat complex, difficult orthodontic cases effectively.

Orthodontics is concerned with the treatment of *malocclusions*. A malocclusion occurs when a patient has teeth that are positioned improperly. In other words, the teeth do not fit together correctly when the jaws are closed. This may occur because the teeth are improperly positioned within one or both jaws; or because the jaws may not be comparable in size.

Malocclusions may cause deformities of the face and/or jaws (e.g., protruding front teeth). Deformities of the face and/or jaws, however, may also result in malocclusions (e.g. cleft palate). If the jaws are mismatched, an orthodontist will occasionally work with an oral and maxillofacial surgeon (another dental specialist) to correct the improper position or size of the jaws in order to change the structure and appearance of the face.

Several studies published in the professional literature on malocclusions have indicated that 50 percent of the population needs some form of orthodontic care. Some malocclusions are hereditary and can be handed down for generations. Hereditary causes include: extra or congenitally missing teeth, misaligned jaws, and teeth with too little or too much space between them. Problems can also occur if the relationship between jaw and teeth size is not proportional. Malocclusions can also be acquired. The causes include: early loss of teeth because of advanced decay or an accident; sucking habits, e.g. thumb or finger sucking; tongue thrusting; improper biting habits, e.g. lip biting; retention of baby teeth; and mouth breathing (which dries out the delicate gum tissue and causes it to be red and inflammed). In addition, some authorities feel that certain sleeping postures can produce pressure on the jaws and effect occlusion.

The same advantages and considerations that apply to child orthodontics also apply to adult orthodontics. In both instances, the orthodontic treatment is done to improve tooth position. The same tissue (bone) is involved in treating an orthodontic patient regardless of the age. Bone readily responds to the force of pressure. Therefore, pressure on the teeth from orthodontics brings about changes in the bone that results in the repositioning of teeth. Treatment may take a little longer for adults because their facial bones have stopped growing. Certain orthodontic corrections require a combination of surgery with conventional orthodontics. Dramatic facial changes in adults have been achieved with this team approach.

There are some inconveniences during orthodontic treatment. For example, there is initial discomfort from sore teeth when the orthodontic braces are placed on the teeth. Additional discomfort is usually experienced when the braces are periodically adjusted. Usually, there is also a feeling of self-consciousness. Braces can initially make talking or even chewing difficult. It takes perseverance and dedication to be an orthodontic patient. You must cooperate fully with your orthodontist to be sure that your (and his) goal is attained.

The benefits of orthodontics include having a healthier mouth. Your teeth have a better chance of lasting a lifetime if they are placed in good alignment. This makes them easier to keep clean. Well-aligned teeth also give you an improved facial appearance. With this comes increased self-esteem. Teeth have to be in proper alignment for you to be able to bite off and chew nutritious, high-fiber foods well enough to be digested easily. A poor bite can also cause extra stress on the chewing muscles, which can result in pain or problems with the joints in the jaw. Protruding teeth are more easily chipped or fractured. Malocclusion can cause abnormal wear on the tooth surfaces.

Orthodontic treatment time depends on the complexity of the treatment needs. Factors to consider are: the severity of the malocclusion; the health of the teeth, gums, and supporting bone; the age of the patient; and the compliance level of the patient. With full compliance, active treatment can last from a few months to two or more years. But even after active orthodontic treatment is completed, you will need to see the orthodontist periodically to maintain the teeth in their new positions. You may need to wear a *retainer* (a removable appliance to keep the teeth in proper position) for a period of time after the appliances are removed.

The cost you might encounter for orthodontics depends on the time required for treatment. This is directly related to the severity of your problem. The only way to determine the cost is to consult your orthodontist.

You might be interested in knowing that the cost of orthodontics has not risen as rapidly as the cost of other dental, or even medical, care. There are many dental insurance companies that will help pay for orthodontics, thus reducing the out-of-pocket cost to you.

To determine your particular orthodontic needs, the orthodontist will probably take a complete medical/dental health history, perform a clinical examination, make models (replicas of your teeth in plaster), take X-ray films of your teeth and head, and take color photographs of your face and teeth. Orthodontists usually take special X-ray films called lateral head X-ray films to determine your present facial profile and tooth position. Using these diagnostic tools, the orthodontist can develop a treatment plan outlining the best course of action for your needs.

If orthodontics is necessary, the "usual" or fixed braces are attached to the teeth in two ways. First, orthodontic *bands* may be cemented to the teeth. Then an *arch wire* is attached to the bands. Tightening the arch wire puts tension on the teeth. The tension gradually moves the teeth to their proper location.

Second, fixed braces may involve bonding *brackets* to the front of the teeth. Like orthodontic bands, arch wires can also be attached to the brackets. A bracket is a tiny plate that can be metal, clear, or tooth-colored. To make these tooth-colored brackets even more esthetic, thinner wires are available so they are less noticeable. The technology of today has now made available *"space age" wires*. They shorten the overall treatment time and the amount of discomfort after adjustments. These wires are made of a super-elastic material (nickel-titanium) that exerts steady, gentle pressure on the teeth.

As previously stated, orthodontic brackets or bands with arch wires are at the heart of moving teeth to their proper positions within a dental arch. Proper alignment within the dental arch, the upper or lower teeth, is primarily attained by stresses on the teeth exerted by an arch wire. In addition, rubber bands (called *elastics* by your orthodontist) are attached to these orthodontic appliances to aid in obtaining the proper tooth alignment. White-colored elastics that blend in with the teeth are available for those patients who are more esthetically conscious (usually adults). Younger patients often prefer the new brightly colored elastics that are now available. The elastics direct the forces of the arch wires.

The elastic exerts its force when it is stretched and the more it is stretched, the greater the force. Thus, the effectiveness of elastics is dependent upon active forces.

Most patients remove the elastics while they are eating. Otherwise they cannot chew properly. Sometimes orthodontic patients forget to replace the elastics, or they lose or run out of them. Additionally, the elastics deteriorate during use and must be changed frequently. For effective treatment in orthodontics the patient must cooperate. It cannot be overemphasized that conscientious and consistent cooperation is the only road to successful treatment. This is a time when the results you achieve are directly dependent upon the effort you put into your treatment.

If a wire on your appliance causes irritation, cover the end with a small cotton ball or beeswax until you can get to the dentist. If the wire gets stuck in the cheek, tongue, or gum tissue, do not try to remove it yourself. Call your dentist immediately. If an appliance becomes loose or breaks off, take the appliance and any broken pieces with you to the dentist as soon as possible so it can be repaired.

Have your child checked by an orthodontist by the age of seven if there is any question about the possible necessity of orthodontic treatment. It is at this age that the permanent teeth begin to replace the *deciduous* teeth (or "baby teeth"). An early examination allows the orthodontist to determine when the problem should be treated for maximum results with the least time and expense.

Orthodontic treatment can begin at any age. However, in some cases early treatment allows results to be attained that could not be achieved after the face and jaws have finished growing. Sometimes it is possible to minimize children's orthodontic problems by doing interceptive orthodontic treatment. This means heading off the problem before it becomes severe and requires extensive treatment at a later stage in your child's development. Interceptive care can often be done by your general dentist, who is trained to help prevent orthodontic problems and to treat simple irregularities in tooth position.

The decision of who should be treating a case is sometimes very controversial. It is important to realize that orthodontics is a branch of dentistry that *can* be practiced by a general dentist, but it may not be in your best interest to have a general dentist do the treatment. The experience level and training between the general dentist and an orthodontist obviously differs; and therefore, the quality of care delivered can also be expected to differ. The best advice I can give is that you consult with an orthodontist if you feel you or a family member needs orthodontic treatment. It could be the best money you have ever spent. The orthodontist can then contact your general dentist to coordinate how the general dentist will be involved with the orthodontic treatment.

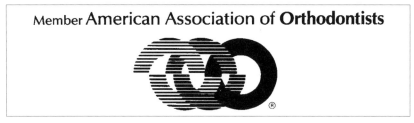

Figure 6

One way of locating a dentist with the proper credentials is to write to: The American Association of Orthodontists (AAO), 460 N. Lindbergh Blvd., St. Louis, Missouri 63141. Or you may phone toll free at: 1-800-STRAIGHT (787-2444); or call non–toll free at 1-314-993-1700.

If you write or call the American Association of Orthodontists, ask for their "Orthodontic Planning Kit." It contains information on low-cost orthodontic/dental insurance and a listing of trained, recognized orthodontists close to your home (usually sent in the form of orthodontists who reside within a specific mailing zip code).

One other way of checking if your dentist is a board-eligible orthodontist is to look for the AAO logo (figure 6). Members of the AAO exhibit this logo. This is true even in Canada.

Now let us see how to determine if you or your child needs orthodontics and what benefits you can get from it.

HOW TO KNOW IF YOU OR YOUR CHILD NEEDS BRACES

If you or your child does not have a nice smile because of crooked teeth, orthodontics can probably solve all or part of the problem. Orthodontics not only can help straighten your teeth but it also can help keep your self-esteem and self-confidence intact by improving your appearance. This will impact both your personal and your business relationships. Speech can also be affected by a severe malocclusion, and this is another critical reason to have the problem treated.

Unusual tooth position, as overlapping or crowded teeth, can result in increased dental decay (caries), premature tooth wear, and discomfort on biting. The results can be difficulty performing proper dental home care (e.g. brushing and flossing) and premature tooth loss.

The consequences of teeth that do not bite together properly can be soreness to either the teeth involved or to the *temporomandibular joint*

(TMJ). This is the hinge joint connecting the lower jaw to the upper jaw. Localized soreness of a tooth caused by improper tooth position may be corrected to a *limited* extent by *occlusal equilibration*. This means that the tooth can be ground by your dentist into properly balanced *occlusion* with the adjacent teeth. But this is similar to taking an aspirin for a brain tumor. The source of the problem is not resolved. On a more generalized level, poor occlusion can lead to headaches, neckaches, sore teeth, and facial pain. This pathological entity has been technically termed *temporomandibular disorder* (TMD). More about this will be discussed later.

Here is a check list of some indicators for anyone who feels he might need orthodontic treatment. These problems affect both the appearance and the function of teeth.

1. Perhaps the first thing that comes to mind when an orthodontist is mentioned is "buck" teeth. This could be caused by thumbsucking or tongue thrusting (pushing against the teeth with the tongue during swallowing). Orthodontists refer to this malocclusion as *upper protrusion*. Not correcting this condition can cause mouth breathing, periodontal disease, and possibly lung infections.
2. The outer surfaces of the upper teeth should slightly overlie the outer surfaces of the lower teeth when the teeth bite together normally. If this proper relationship does not exist, the malocclusion is called a *crossbite*. This is sometimes most pronounced in the front teeth. Usually, a person with this problem will have a frowning expression.
3. The midline between the upper and lower central incisors should line up. When this does not occur, it is technically termed a *misplaced midline*.
4. Teeth should work as a unit. Proper function is lost if there is space between the biting surfaces of either the front or side teeth when the back teeth bite together. This is called an *open bite*. Not correcting this condition can result in gingival or periodontal disease.
5. Sometimes the upper front teeth lie too far over the lower front teeth. It can be so severe that the lower teeth bite into the roof of the mouth. Not correcting this *overbite* can result in periodontal disease.
6. An *underbite* or "bulldog" appearance occurs when either the lower teeth are too far in front or the upper teeth are too far back.
7. *Spacing* may be the result of congenitally missing teeth, extracted teeth, or small teeth. Essentially, there is too much dental ridge to accommodate either the number or the size of the teeth. This spacing allows food to be trapped between the teeth. When there are too many teeth for the dental ridge to accommodate it is called *crowded teeth*. If not corrected, both of these conditions will result in periodontal disease.

If you detect any of these problems I would recommend that you see an orthodontist for a consultation. A decision can be made after considering the cost versus the benefits that you or your child can derive from orthodontic treatment.

It is easiest to have orthodontics done as a child or young adult, but orthodontics may be done at any time in a person's life. In fact, *adult orthodontics* is becoming more and more in vogue. Many adults are now undergoing orthodontic treatment because their families could not afford it when they were young. It may take a longer period of time and be somewhat more complicated to achieve results as an adult in treatment. In orthodontics, it is seldom, if ever, too late to seek treatment.

ESTHETIC BRACES

Braces of the nineties are "cool looking." It is no longer necessary to tolerate the nickname "brace face" or "metal mouth." Braces today are smaller, lighter, and show far less metal than in the past. In fact, one of the latest fads is colored braces. Wearing braces that are hot pink, purple, blue, or grape can even be fun. Braces now have scaled-down "mini" brackets that bond to the front teeth, which eliminates the need for bands. Some braces offer plastic-coated wires in either white or ivory color. Another option is transparent or tooth-colored bracketed braces with thinner wires. These braces bond directly to the front teeth. Strides in recent years in wire technology have made available both clear, fiber-optic, and Teflon-coated arch wires for more pleasing esthetics. Orthodontists now use super-elastic, braided, shape-memory arch wires to correct malocclusions without unesthetic bends in the wires that show in the front of the mouth.

Fixed esthetic braces (also known as lingual braces) are placed on the tongue side of the teeth, making them "invisible" because they cannot be seen from the front. The brackets are cemented to the backs of the front teeth as far back as the bicuspids. Then the arch wire is attached to the brackets. This differs from "conventional" braces, which are placed on the fronts of the teeth. Placing the brackets on the back of the teeth causes the forces that affect tooth movement to work by pulling rather than pushing the teeth into proper position.

The disadvantage of these braces is they are sometimes irritating to the tongue and cause speech difficulties; they are more expensive because they are difficult to place and control and require more frequent visits; and they cannot be used in some types of malocclusion because placement of the brackets would not allow the patient to put his teeth together. If you have any interest in this approach to orthodontic treatment you should discuss it with your orthodontist.

Some removable appliances (braces) are held in place by clasps that fit over selected teeth. Other removable appliances use straps that fit on your head. There is nothing new about these concepts. Orthodontists use such removable appliances as retainers to help keep the teeth in their new location after fixed braces have been removed.

Appliances that can be removed during times involving public contact have recently gained a lot of publicity. This eliminates the usual braces that must be worn during the entire active treatment. Though some patients are attracted to this approach, there is a problem. The American Association of Orthodontists states that when using the removable appliances "it is almost always necessary to complete treatment with conventional braces."

Removable appliances do have a place in orthodontic treatment. Instead of applying pressure directly to teeth as conventional braces do, removable appliances are used both to change the structure of the jaws and/or face and to retain (with a retainer) repositioned teeth. The retainer keeps the teeth in their new correct positions until the tissues surrounding them stabilize. It is important to remember that removable appliances may be used either before or after conventional braces are placed, but they are very seldom used instead of conventional braces.

7

Pediatric Dentistry

A pediatric dentist is a specialist in children's dental care and in the growth and development of children's facial structure and teeth. The most current definition of pediatric dentistry (once called pedodontics) endorsed by the American Academy of Pediatric Dentistry is: "An age-defined specialty that provides both primary and specialty comprehensive preventive and therapeutic oral health care for infants and children through adolescence, including those with special health care needs."

General dentists are licensed to take care of most dental problems your child might have. The decision whether to take your child to a general dentist or to a pediatric dentist is quite similar to one's choice of a physician in family medicine or in pediatrics. The pediatric dentist has had two years extra training beyond dental school in a recognized ADA training program. He is very familiar with the growth and development of children as it relates to their dental health. Thus, with their specialty training, they have the ability to pick up a dental-related problem your child may have that might be overlooked by a general dentist who has not had special training. He also is trained to manage children to insure that their dental experience is positive.

On occasion, a child may have medical or emotional problems, handicaps, a complex treatment plan, or patient management problems. In these instances, your child would probably most benefit from the expertise of the pediatric dentist.

Usually pediatric dental offices are furnished with tables, chairs, wall decorations, etc. that are geared for children. They also have dental equipment that is smaller so the dentists can more easily accommodate the small mouths of children.

111
▲

Currently, many pediatric dentists recommend that children start their dental visits when the first primary teeth erupt (between six and twelve months of age). Pediatric dentists feel this is the first of three "milestones" they have identified as important to monitor in early child development. At this first milestone you can get very valuable information from your dentist concerning tooth development, the need for fluoride, how to help a child maintain proper dental hygiene, how to deal with your child's oral habits (e.g. pacifier use), diet and nutrition, and how to prevent oral injuries. Identifying dental problems before they become advanced is the key to preventing costly and painful treatments in the future.

It is precisely at this time that the dentist can be your most valuable resource as your child's oral health adviser. For example, one potential problem that you should be warned about at this time is called *baby bottle syndrome*. This condition is caused by frequent exposure of a child's teeth for long periods of time to liquids containing sugars, e.g. milk, formula, fruit juice, etc. The teeth most frequently damaged are the upper front teeth. Thus, instead of offering your child a bottle containing any of the above sugars during their nap times, fill the bottle with water or give the child a pacifier recommended by your dentist or physician. During sleep, the flow of saliva decreases, allowing the liquids in the nursing bottle to pool around the child's teeth for long periods. After each feeding, wipe your baby's teeth and gums with a clean, damp washcloth or gauze pad. It is also important to let your dentist know at this time of early development if your water supply does not contain fluoride so he can provide you with a prescription so it can be added to the bottle.

Teeth start to erupt at about six months of age and continue until age three. This causes many children to have tender gums and become irritable. It helps to rub the gums with your finger, a small cool spoon, or a teething ring (many can be put in the freezer so they are more soothing). Most health professionals will tell you it is not normal to have a fever while teething. However, many mothers will tell you it is quite common! If your baby has a fever when teething, it is best to contact your physician to rule out the possibility that the child has some other problem.

Your child's first dental experience should be a pleasant one. Pediatric dentists and experienced general dentists have found that the best approach is not to rush the child through treatment. In fact, your child's first dental visit will most likely be nothing more than an introduction to the dentist (and perhaps his hygienist): the child will sit in the dental chair, handle and touch the dental instruments, and see how the chair goes up and down and tilts back. The dentist may count the teeth of a cooperative child. Even though treatment may not be performed at the early visits, it gives the dentist a chance to study the child's dental growth and development. This is important!

A second milestone when your dentist will want to see your child is between 12 and 24 months of age. This is the time when the primary teeth have erupted, relationships between upper and lower teeth are established, and the arch length has been determined.

Yet another milestone occurs from two to six years of age. It is during this time the first primary teeth are lost and the first permanent molars or incisors have erupted. With an extremely cooperative patient, X-ray films are sometimes done at these early visits.

Nonnutritive sucking (thumb sucking) should be addressed in this milestone. Sucking is a natural reflex that makes young children feel secure and happy in difficult periods, as when they are separated from their parents or disciplined. Since it is relaxing, it is often done when tired or at night to induce sleep. This habit can cause problems with the growth of the mouth and alignment of the teeth, if it continues after the permanent teeth have erupted. It can also cause changes in the roof of the mouth. Studies show the intensity of the sucking affects the degree of the problems that occur as a result of thumb sucking.

Most authorities agree thumb sucking should cease by the time the permanent front teeth are ready to erupt. Children usually stop this habit between two and four years of age. If the habit continues, peer pressure causes many school age children to stop because the behavior is viewed negatively by classmates. Many times children who still have this habit after entering school have more problems making friends. Sucking pacifiers causes essentially the same affect as thumb sucking. However, it is usually easier to break a pacifier sucking habit. Older children should be involved in the choice of method used to stop this habit. Rather than scold children for sucking, authorities encourage parents to use positive reinforcement and praise children when they are not sucking. Parents should focus on correcting the cause of the anxiety in the child that is causing him to suck. If the child is sucking for comfort, provide it and reward the child when he refrains from sucking during difficult periods. It is sometimes helpful to remind the child of the habit by bandaging the thumb or putting a sock on the hand at night. Bitter medication can be prescribed by your dentist or pediatrician to coat the thumb or an appliance to use in the mouth can be fabricated.

The reason for regular visits in the early years is to monitor oral development. It is important not to frighten the child by introducing too many new experiences too rapidly. These first introductions to the dentist must be pleasant to insure that he has a positive image of dentistry and the dentist in the future. Never threaten a child with seeing the dentist as a punishment or say to him how sorry you are he has to go to the dentist. *Always emphasize a dental visit as a positive experience.* Explain to your child that visiting the dentist helps maintain good oral health. In addition, starting visits to the dentist early and continuing them at regular six-month intervals helps to give your child a positive attitude toward regular care. This positive attitude will last a lifetime, in most instances.

Most dentists prefer to see young patients in the morning when they are rested. Never make an appointment that will conflict with the child's mealtimes or nap.

After each visit, the dentist should discuss his findings and subsequently proposed treatment (if needed) of your child with you, the parent. The dentist should also discuss with you your child's necessary home care; what your child should be eating and how his eating habits can influence his future dental health; what fluoride supplements may be necessary; and what future visits and care may be needed.

Counting your child's teeth as they erupt and noting the time of eruption is one of the most important dental services you can perform for your child. The lower four incisors are usually the first "baby" teeth to erupt. These same four teeth are the first to be shed, making way for the adult teeth. The following is a chart for reference in checking your child's tooth eruption and shedding.

Your child should have twenty "baby teeth" by about the age of two years. Check with your dentist if this is not the case. By checking, you can prevent problems that could be very costly to correct later in your child's life.

Since pediatric dentists are specialists in growth and development, your child should be examined by one if he or she has teeth that are not

ERUPTION AND SHEDDING OF "BABY" TEETH

Upper	Eruption	Shedding
Central incisor	8–12 mos.	6–7 yrs.
Lateral incisor	9–13 mos.	7–8 yrs.
Cuspid	16–22 mos.	10–12 yrs.
First molar	13–19 mos.	9–11 yrs.
Second molar	25–33 mos.	10–12 yrs.

Lower	Eruption	Shedding
Central incisor	6–10 mos.	6–7 yrs.
Lateral incisor	10–16 mos.	7–8 yrs.
Cuspid	17–23 mos.	9–12 yrs.
First molar	14–18 mos.	9–11 yrs.
Second molar	23–31 mos.	10–12 yrs.

ERUPTION OF ADULT TEETH

Upper	Eruption
Central incisor	7–8 yrs.
Lateral incisor	8–9 yrs.
Cuspid	11–12 yrs.
First bicuspid	10–11 yrs.
Second bicuspid	10–12 yrs.
First molar	6–7 yrs.
Second molar	12–13 yrs.
Third molar	17–21 yrs.

Lower	Eruption
Central incisor	6–7 yrs.
Lateral incisor	7–8 yrs.
Cuspid	9–10 yrs.
First bicuspid	10–12 yrs.
Second bicuspid	11–12 yrs.
First molar	6–7 yrs.
Second molar	11–13 yrs.
Third molar	17–21 yrs.

erupting according to the above schedule (or near it), or if your child has physical or emotional limitations. The next section of this chapter will explain more in depth why "baby teeth" are important.

WHY ARE "BABY" TEETH IMPORTANT?

It is not always clear to parents why "baby teeth" (or, more accurately, *deciduous* teeth) should not be extracted. These teeth begin to erupt at about six months. But the child retains them until he or she is about 11 or 12 years of age. That is well beyond the baby stage. The deciduous teeth guide the adult teeth into their proper position. The loss of a deciduous tooth earlier than nature intended is the loss of the adult tooth's guide for proper positioning; hence, the tooth will likely come in crooked or in the wrong place in the dental arch. The child may require orthodontic treatment to straighten these teeth. Waiting to correct the situation when the child is older can be both more time consuming and more costly than when early intervention occurs.

Most of the orthodontists I surveyed estimated that premature loss of deciduous teeth is the reason why orthodontic treatment is needed in at least 30 percent of the cases. So save those deciduous teeth. If it does become necessary to remove a deciduous tooth, talk to your dentist about taking measures to keep the space open where the deciduous tooth is located until the permanent tooth erupts. In other words, it is necessary to keep the other teeth in the mouth from drifting into the space where a deciduous tooth has been removed. Otherwise, the permanent tooth will not be able to erupt into the space where the deciduous tooth was located. Decay and possible loss of deciduous teeth can cause loss of appetite, as well as being unhealthy for your child. Hot, cold, or hard foods may be more difficult for the child to eat. Difficulty with speech or loss of self-esteem are additional problems.

The pediatric dentists I surveyed stated that in the first few appointments a dentist should spend time not only in "fixing" your child's teeth, but also in studying the youngster's dental growth and development.

If you get nothing else from this chapter, please note this last statement. Studying and understanding your child's growth and development is the key to preventing problems that might otherwise make orthodontic treatment necessary in the future. Dentists should save teeth; but they should not overlook the bigger picture . . . the future dental picture.

The dentist to whom you take your child should be made aware of your own daily observations of your child's behavior. Tell him about thumb sucking, tongue-thrusting habits during swallowing or speaking, or enlarged tonsils or adenoids. Your pediatrician might also be able to offer you some insights into some of the above information.

Finally, the ADA sponsors a national campaign called Children's Dental Health Month during February each year. The campaign is to encourage youngsters and their parents to be more conscious of children's dental health. During Children's Dental Health Month, individual dentists from many of the various state dental organizations donate their time to screen and educate kids and their parents about their children's dental care. New continuing education pamphlets are constantly being printed for parents to help make them more knowledgable about their child's dental health. It is very important for parents to motivate their children to have good oral health. Most of these educational materials can be obtained from your general dentist or pediatric dentist. In addition, the ADA will send you a free copy of each of their pamphlets on a particular topic or one copy of all the pamphlets they have available for distribution by writing directly to the ADA, Bureau of Health and Audiovisual Services, 211 E. Chicago Avenue, Chicago, Illinois 60611.

There are no excuses for being an uninformed parent. Your child's teeth depend on it.

SEALANTS

New guidelines recommend the use of sealants for both adults and children who are at risk of pit-and-fissure caries (decay). A sealant is a clear or shaded plastic material that is applied to the chewing surfaces of the back teeth (premolars and molars). Since this is where decay occurs most often, the sealant acts as a barrier to protect the decay-prone areas of the back teeth from plaque and acid. Studies have shown that 85 percent of the dental caries occurs on the chewing surfaces of the back teeth. Fluoride has practically eliminated caries on the smooth surfaces of the biting teeth (the teeth located in the front of the mouth). Pit-and-fissure sealants have been fully approved by the ADA since 1976. At this writing, we are using third-generation materials that are cured by visible light.

Because of irregularities on the chewing surfaces of the teeth, it is impossible for the patient to keep then clean because the bristles of the toothbrush cannot reach into them. Thus, trapped food particles and bacteria in these areas often result in dental caries. Sealants form a thin covering over the irregularities of the pits and fissures of the teeth, keeping out plaque and food and resulting in a decrease in the incidence of caries in these areas.

The method of application is simple. First, the teeth that will be sealed are cleaned by the dental professional. Then, a mild acidic solution is applied to the chewing surfaces to etch (roughen) them to help the sealants adhere to the teeth. Finally, the sealant is brushed on the tooth and allowed to harden. Some sealants need a special curing light to help them harden. Sealants need to be inspected each time patients return for their regular dental visit. It usually takes several years before reapplication of the sealant is necessary. The average cost ranges from $10 to $40 per tooth, depending on the particular case.

Children benefit most from sealants applied to their teeth, especially to newly erupted permanent teeth. Continued reapplication of sealants through the adult years has been shown to be a valuable method for decreasing the incidence of caries in the adult population. Authorities feel that the combined use of sealants with systemic and topical application of fluorides throughout life, periodic dental checkups, eating a limited amount of sugar-rich foods, and daily brushing and flossing will eliminate caries in the near future.

Surveys show that despite attempts by health agencies to promote sealants, the utilization rates are still low. The reason is because of misconceptions about their effectiveness and a lack of awareness about sealants. It will make a dramatic difference if the children who are poor, without dental insurance, and do not see the dentist very often are given access to sealants. One of the oral health objectives of the U.S. Public Health Service's Healthy People 2000 project is that 50 percent of American children have sealants on their teeth by the year 2000.

TETRACYCLINES AND YOUR CHILD'S TEETH

Parents should be aware that the tetracyclines, a group of frequently prescribed antibiotics, can cause tooth discoloration. More than 2,000 patents for different members of this group of antibiotics have been issued since they were first introduced to medicine in 1948.

Tetracyclines have been used for medical problems ranging from lung and urinary infections to acne. They are frequently used in dentistry to treat periodontitis and some forms of gingivitis. Sometimes they are used for the treatment of abscessed teeth.

These antibiotics are safe and effective, but they come with the following warning: Tetracyclines should not be used by nursing mothers or by expectant mothers during the last half of pregnancy. In addition, they should not be prescribed to children age eight or younger. Most physicians recognize this concern.

Be sure to tell your physician or dentist if you are a new mother who is still nursing because the antibiotic will pass on to the baby through your milk. The amount of tetracycline passed to the infant from nursing can cause tooth discoloration.

Tetracyclines, in very rare instances, could be necessary to save your child's life or even your own life. Tooth discoloration is a very small price to pay for a life. But, medical authorities say, a nursing mother can take measures before taking tetracyclines to prevent damage to her child's teeth. She should stop nursing while taking the tetracycline and not resume until 48 hours after the last dose is taken. This allows time for the antibiotic to be cleared from the mother's system.

The degree and nature of tooth discoloration from tetracyclines depends on many factors. These include the dosage, the duration of the medication, the type of tetracycline used, and the point of tooth development when the antibiotic was given.

Exactly how tetracyclines cause tooth discoloration is well documented. In simple terms, the tetracycline combines with the calcium in the developing tooth and becomes part of the tooth structure. The only benefit (if you want to call it that) is that these discolored teeth seem to be more resistant to dental decay than non-stained teeth.

Medical authorities say that self-medication with "saved-up" drugs probably accounts for most tetracycline staining today. Nursing mothers who are unaware of the hazards sometimes take the antibiotics without the knowledge of their physician or dentist.

Do not save old tetracyclines! Not only could they harm your child's teeth, but they also could make you (or your child) very ill. If the pills have passed the expiration date on the prescription bottle, throw them out. Tetracyclines, unlike other antibiotics which simply lose their potency, become *toxic* (poisonous) after their expiration date.

INJURY TO YOUR CHILD'S TEETH

"Mom, I fell off my bike and knocked out one of my front teeth. What should I do?" Billy is standing in the doorway, crying and bleeding. This is one of those instances when fear often turns to panic for mothers.

The ADA estimates that by the time young adults graduate from high school, one in three boys and one in four girls have experienced some type of traumatic injury to their teeth. Such injuries can result from falls, auto accidents, contact sports, or any number of other causes.

Essentially there are four types of tooth injuries, with some subcategories. The basic types are as follows:

1. *Luxation.* A tooth injury in which the tooth has sustained a blow. The tooth may not have been displaced in its socket, in which case it is termed a concussion injury. In a displacement injury a blow has loosened the tooth but not to the point of knocking it out.
2. *Avulsion.* The tooth has been entirely knocked out of the socket.
3. *Intrusion.* The tooth has been pushed up farther into the socket as a result of the blow.
4. *Fracture.* The tooth has been broken. A crown fracture involves a break only in the part of the tooth above the gums. Crown fractures may range from a minor chip (this includes 90 percent of all injuries) to an exposure of the pulp (the central part of the tooth). A root fracture is a break somewhere in the root portion of the tooth (tooth structure below the gum line).

The rule to follow if you or your child has one of these injuries is to contact your dentist (either general dentist or the appropriate specialist) as soon as possible. Even a small chip that can apparently just be smoothed down could result in the death of the pulp. In other words, you could end up with an abscessed tooth. In fact, a tooth in which the crown has sustained a hard blow without fracturing is more likely to abscess than one in which the root has fractured.

If a permanent tooth is avulsed (knocked out), the key to successful replantation is to get the tooth reimplanted in the socket as soon as possible. With each minute that passes more of the cells on the root of the tooth die. These cells are needed to attach the root back in the socket. Whenever possible the tooth should be reimplated at the site and the patient taken to the dentist as soon as possible. However, many times the patient is frightened and uncooperative, so the tooth cannot be reimplanted. If the tooth has to be transported to the dentist for reimplantation, it is important to pick it up only by the crown and put it in a transport medium. If it is dirty, it can be rinsed gently, but take care not to injure the root of the tooth where the cells for attachment are located. If you are in a situation that requires you to get a tooth reimplanted, it is important to never do any of the following: scrub or brush the root surface, use soap or chemicals to clean the tooth, dry the tooth, or wrap the tooth in a tissue or cloth! The most suitable medium to use to transport the tooth is Hank's Balanced Salt Solution (HBSS), a mammalian tissue culture medium that can be purchased over the counter in most local drugstores. Ideally, this solution would be readily available in a small container at the site of the accident or in family first aid kits. The next best medium to use to transport the tooth is milk, followed by saline, saliva from the side of the cheek, or water. *The key point is that the tooth must not be allowed to dry!* The best chance for success is reimplantation within the first thirty minutes, with chances still considered very good up to the first two hours. To get the most favorable results, root canal therapy should be started one to two weeks after the tooth has been stabilized.

If the tooth is loose or has been knocked out and replaced in its socket, the dentist will most likely want to stabilize it. This is done by temporarily attaching the loose tooth to the adjacent teeth, a process called *splinting*. In cases where the tooth is loose but has not come out of the socket, the splint is usually left in place seven to ten days, or until mobility is within acceptable limits. While a tooth is in a splint, it is important to avoid biting on it, eat soft foods, and maintain good oral hygiene.

In cases where the tooth is fractured (broken), the injured area should be cleaned with warm water. If cold compresses are placed on the face in the area of the injured tooth it will help decrease the swelling. You must see your dentist as soon as possible!

If you get objects (bone, food, etc.) caught between teeth, it is best to try to remove them with floss. Don't ever try to remove anything that is between your teeth with a sharp or pointed instrument. If you are not successful, go to your dentist.

If you have a toothache, be sure to rinse with warm water and use dental floss to remove food particles. This is often the source of the pain.

Never place an aspirin on the aching tooth or gum tissue because that will burn it. However, it is all right to swallow an analgesic (ibuprofen or aspirin). If there is swelling present, you need to begin taking antibiotics as soon as possible. Never put hot compresses on a swollen face because it will make the swelling worse. If you are not able to reach your dentist and the swelling or pain seems to be increasing at a rapid rate, you should go to the nearest emergency room for an evaluation and treatment. They can provide an antibiotic and pain medication injection that will begin working immediately. Severe pain and swelling should not be taken lightly. Make an appointment with your dentist as soon as possible!

If you suspect you or someone you know has a broken jaw, do not move it. The jaw should be secured in place with a handkerchief, necktie, or towel that is tied around the jaw and over the top of the head. Cold compresses should be used to control swelling, if present. Go immediately to a hospital emergency room, or call your dentist.

After any type of blow to the teeth, the major cause of tooth loss in *root resorption*. This means the root of the tooth slowly dissolves away through bodily processes. This is similar to the mechanism involved in the roots of "baby teeth" when they resorb (dissolve) and become loose. The possibility of root resorption is one of the main reasons that the dentist should keep track of the injured tooth with X rays taken at intervals no longer than six months.

If your dentist sees resorption occurring, there are techniques that can halt the process and save the tooth. This includes the placement of calcium hydroxide in the root canal space of the resorbing tooth. It will then be necessary to return to the dentist in three to eight weeks for root canal therapy.

Studies show that after a root fracture about 80 percent of the teeth maintain healthy pulps. The other injuries described above result in almost certain pulp death, resulting in the need for root canal therapy.

In summary, get your child or yourself to your dentist as soon as possible after an injury to a tooth. It is also important to have frequent, regular checkups on the injured tooth to prevent its loss from root resorption. Most teeth, even those with fractured roots or those that have been totally knocked out, can be saved with proper care.

MOUTH GUARDS

Studies show that intraoral mouth guards protect players against injuries to the teeth and lips, and reduce the chances of serious injury to the head and neck areas such as concussions and jaw fractures. When a mouth guard is in place, it is less likely the person will sustain chipped or fractured teeth, nerve damage, or tooth loss. Oral injuries are not uncommon among athletes. However, because mouth guards are mandatory, football players do not usually sustain oral injuries. Therefore, most authorities feel athletes in all sports should wear mouth guards—even if it is not mandatory. In fact, many feel that any child who is participating in an activity that involves falls, head contact, tooth clenching, or flying equipment (anything from basketball, skateboarding to gymnastics to soccer) should wear a mouth guard.

The three types of mouth guards available are custom made, self-adapted, and stock. Custom-made mouth guards are individually designed and constructed by a dentist or professional laboratory. After an impression of the athlete's teeth is taken, the mouth guard is fabricated over a stone model of the teeth. Usually a mouth guard covers only the upper teeth. Even though custom-made mouth guards are more expensive, they are the most comfortable and the most preferred by athletes. Their good fit and overall quality makes them worth the extra expense. These mouth guards are easily retained in the mouth and do not interfere with speech or breathing. Self-adapted (also called boil and bite) mouth guards come in a preformed shape that can be altered by boiling the mouth guard in water and biting into the warm plastic for a customized fit. Stock mouth guards cannot be altered except to trim excess material from the edges. They fit loosely over the teeth.

One recent study determined that the oral injury rate for athletes who wore mouth guards was 2.8 percent and the oral injury rate for those not wearing mouth guards was 30.3 percent. Studies have further concluded that athletes prefer the most comfortable mouth guard and will wear it more often and longer. This offers more protection for the athlete. Mouth guards need to be replaced after each sports season. Many athletes who play several sports have new mouth guards fabricated when they go for their six-month checkup.

8

Periodontics

Periodontics is an ADA-recognized specialty that involves the study of the causes, prevention, diagnosis, and treatment of diseases of the supportive tissues of the teeth. Supportive tissues, which include the gingiva (gum) and the underlying bone, hold the teeth in the upper and lower jaws. An ADA-recognized specialist in periodontics is called a periodontist. He must complete a two-year, ADA-approved training program beyond dental school before he can list himself as a specialist in periodontics.

Periodontal (gum) disease is defined as inflammation of the gingiva and the adjacent supporting structures of the teeth. The ADA estimates over half of all adults over the age of 18 have at least the primary stages of periodontal disease. Since this disease usually does not cause severe pain, it many times goes unnoticed.

Researchers have recently reported a profile to identify individuals most likely at high risk for periodontal disease. Many authorities feel genetic predisposition to periodontal disease is a factor to consider in individuals. African Americans are four times more susceptible to localized periodontal disease than Asians and 40 times more than Caucasian Americans. A recent Canadian study cross-referenced age with such variables as educational level, income, overall health, and stress. The conclusion was individuals 75 years or older were most likely to have severe periodontal disease. Although periodontal disease has long been associated with systemic diseases (e.g. AIDS, anemia, diabetes), a recent report concluded those individuals who had minimal calculus also were at minimal risk for periodontitis. Calculus and plaque contribute to the progression of periodontal disease rather than its initiation. At this time it is believed certain bacteria in the mouth may be associated with periodontitis, and possibly these certain bacteria may be used in the future to identify high-risk groups for periodontal disease. There is no question smoking and tobacco products contribute to periodontitis. Gingivitis is common during the teen years because of the hormonal changes that occur at this age. Although it more frequently occurs with advancing age, it has even been shown to occur in children as young as five or six years of age. People who practice good oral health care are three times less likely to have periodontal disease. It is very important for those people who are at higher risk for periodontal disease to be more careful to make sure they are taking all the proper precautions at home, and that they are seeing their dentist on a frequently scheduled basis.

Periodontal disease progression is not necessarily continuous, but takes place through acute episodes that alternate with periods of latency. The diagnostic techniques currently available for determining past, present, and the likelihood of future periodontal disease fall into three categories:

1. Clinical techniques for soft tissue evaluation include manual and electronic probing, temperature measurement under the gum tissue, and visual inspection
2. Radiographic techniques for hard tissue evaluation include conventional X rays and filmless digital imaging radiovisiography
3. Microbiological techniques used to test for the presence of bacteria that have been determined to be indicators of periodontal disease.

Since studies confirm that more than 30 percent of periodontal disease is recurrent, it is necessary to identify problem sites regularly before further damage occurs.

NEW TECHNOLOGY FOR DIAGNOSIS OF PERIODONTITIS

All of the traditional tests for periodontal disease (pocket probing, X rays, and visual inspection for inflammation) detect anatomic changes of both hard and soft tissue. The goals of the new microbiological tests, now possible because of technological advances, are to allow early detection of periodontal disease *before* any significant destruction of the bone and connective tissue has occurred. The FDA has recently approved for marketing Periocheck (Prodentec), a test at chairside for elevated levels of specific enzymes that indicate active gingivitis and periodontitis. This has become a very significant part of maintenance for implant patients because it enables *peri-implantitis* (periodontal disease around implants) to be intercepted early in its progression. Recent studies have also correlated an elevated temperature in the pocket of each tooth with current or impending periodontal disease. Currently this can be identified with a PerioTemp (Abioden), a periodontal probe with a thermocouple at the tip to measure temperature changes within the pocket. The temperature is indicated with a red, green, or yellow light, along with a printed copy of the results. The microbiological diagnosis of periodontal disease has advanced at a rapid pace in recent years.

CAUSES AND TREATMENT OF PERIODONTITIS

Periodontal disease is caused by *plaque*, a colorless, sticky film composed of colonies of bacteria that constantly form and attach to the teeth. Of the over 330 types of bacteria that reside in the oral cavity, there are at least 15 different organisms associated with adult periodontitis (gum disease), and some of these same organisms cause dental decay. Studies show that the volume of fluid in the pockets around the tooth correlates with the degree of inflammation of the periodontal disease. Technology now enables testing to be done by collecting a sample of fluid on a paper test strip that is then read by a sensor unit. The traditional method for identifying the bacteria under the gum tissue is sending a bacterial culture to an outside lab for analysis. Identifying the components of the fluid is very useful in diagnosing periodontal disease because this provides information about antibiotic sensitivity of the bacteria when there has been no response to conventional antibiotic therapy. Another useful diagnostic indicator for identifying patients who are at risk for periodontal disease is to identify markers (chemicals that are associated with tissue destruction) in the blood from bleeding gum tissue.

If the plaque is not removed by daily brushing it produces toxins (poisons) that can irritate the gum tissue, causing *gingivitis* (gingival irritation). This early stage of periodontal disease affects only the gum tissue, and at this point it is still reversible. At this stage of the disease, the patient will classically come to the dentist or dental hygienist and report red, swollen, tender gums that bleed whenever they brush.

If the plaque is left undisturbed, the toxins will destroy the underlying bone that holds the teeth in place. As this process occurs, the gingiva may recede away from the crown of the tooth and expose the root surface, causing pockets to form that hold the bacteria on the root surface of the tooth. This may cause the tooth to be sensitive to hot, cold, or biting forces. In addition, the destruction of the bone will cause the teeth to become loose, and eventually the bone loss is so extensive that the teeth will have to be removed. These are signs that the disease has reached the more advanced stage of periodontal disease called *periodontitis*, and at this point it can cause irreversible damage. When these signs and symptoms occur, you should seek immediate attention from your dentist and/or the hygienist.

Tooth brushing removes the plaque, but it should be done properly. Tooth brushing is useless if the plaque has been allowed to harden and become *calculus* or tartar, which can only be removed from your teeth by a dentist or hygienist. Calculus is definitely a contributing factor in periodontal disease. It makes the teeth rough, causing the plaque to be more difficult to remove.

In the advanced stages of periodontal disease the gingiva pulls away from the teeth, and pockets (spaces), which become filled with bacteria and toxins, form around the tooth. These pockets become deeper as the plaque and subsequent calculus continues to collect, and over time the situation becomes more difficult for both the patient and the dentist to manage. If left unattended, periodontal disease may eventually result in the loss of a tooth. In fact, periodontal disease is the primary reason today for tooth loss.

The major cause of periodontal disease is improper preventive care, or simply neglect. "Neglect" implies not getting regular dental check ups and/or not using good tooth brushing and flossing techniques. Periodontal disease can largely be prevented through regular visits to your dentist to have your teeth cleaned and checked, and good home care (including brushing, flossing, etc.). See the home care section of chapter 1 for details.

Another major cause of periodontal disease is smoking and the use of smokeless tobacco. Other factors contributing to periodontal disease include: systemic diseases such as AIDS or diabetes, which can lower the resistence of tissue to infection; unusual hormone levels as occur during pregnancy, which can cause the body to exaggerate any type of reaction to an irritation (even plaque); medications such as those used to control epilepsy, steroids, oral contraceptives, drugs used for treating cancer, or medicines that have a tendency to dry the mouth; poor nutrition; dental conditions such as malocclusions (from the lack of proper orthodontic care), poorly placed fillings that trap food, and poorly fitting *partial dentures* and *bridges*; oral habits such as nail biting, clenching and/or grinding the teeth because of stress; food that becomes impacted between teeth because of improper spacing; and finally, the improper use of toothpicks and floss. Now that is quite a lengthy list of causes. However, it is important to remember these factors do not cause periodontal disease; they only contribute to its severity and risk.

The warning signs of periodontal disease include:

◆ any changes in the way you bite
◆ ill-fitting partial dentures
◆ infection (pus) coming from between or around the gingiva
◆ red, swollen, tender gums that often have pulled away from the teeth
◆ persistent bad breath or bad taste
◆ teeth that are loose or are separating
◆ gums that bleed when you brush your teeth

Most general dentists have a dental hygienist to help patients prevent periodontal disease. For more severe cases, a periodontist is generally called in to assist the general dentist in treating and/or diagnosing complicated diseases of the tissue supporting the tooth.

During checkups, your dentist will examine your gum tissue for periodontal problems. A hand-held instrument called a periodontal probe is traditionally used to determine if there is any breakdown in the attachment of the gingiva or development of pockets between the gingiva and the teeth. The probe has a ruler on its tip so the depth of pockets can be measured. It is generally accepted that pockets 1 to 3 mm are normal, that 4 to 5 mm is moderate pocketing, and that pockets 6 mm or deeper indicate severe trouble. X rays are used to determine the extent of bone that has been destroyed. A disadvantage of these traditional probes has always been that they are extremely operator sensitive due to variations in probing pressure, making the results difficult to reproduce. At this writing there are two electronic constant pressure probes available, and at least two more have been developed for use in research. The microprocessors in these probes provide carefully calibrated probe force, and automatically provide hardcopies of the probing chart for the records. The disadvantages of this new technology are the cost and the increased time required for use. There are also two nonelectronic constant pressure probes on the market that seem to work just as well, and are available at a much more reasonable cost.

The need to have accurate and easily reproducible periodontal charts has led to the development of a number of electronic charting systems. These are stand-alone, computer-generated data collection systems. Some are even voice activated! These systems provide a means to graphically illustrate restorative and periodontal data including bleeding points, recession of the gums, pocket depths, mobility of the teeth, and bone destruction. The charts can even be put into a format on the screen that enables them to be sequentially compared with a patient's previous charts already stored in the computer. We now even have intraoral video cameras and digital imaging radiovisiography (RVG) that interfaces with this software. Many of the digital imaging radiovisiography systems have computer enhancement with colorization to show graphically various stages of periodontal disease.

When periodontal disease is diagnosed patients are treated by using either a non-surgical and/or surgical approach, depending on the stage of advancement of the disease. Nonsurgical periodontal treatment includes scaling and root planing the teeth. *Root planing* involves smoothing the root surface so that plaque will not attach, thus enabling the gingiva to reattach. *Scaling* is the removal of plaque and calculus deposits from root surfaces below the gumline. Usually, when a periodontist cleans teeth, he is cleaning mineral deposits that have accumulated far below the gum line on the root surfaces.

Antibiotics or irrigation with antimicrobials (agents or mouth rinses) are sometimes recommended to help control the growth of bacteria under the gingiva that eventually causes *periodontitis*. Many periodontists use Actisite, a tetracycline-impregnated fiber, as an adjunct in selected cases to scaling and planing to help reduce pocket depth and bleeding when the tissue is probed. The fiber continuously releases tetracycline hydrochloride for 10 days. Even though the levels of tetracycline in the periodontal pocket are constant and 150 times higher than those achieved by oral ingestion, the presence of tetracycline is negligible in the blood. The most common side effects are localized redness after the fiber is removed. Some discomfort on placement of the fiber has also been reported. This treatment has proved successful in localized, active, pockets 5 mm or deeper that have not responded to mechanical therapy. It is necessary to avoid brushing, flossing, or chewing at the treated site during the 10-day course of treatment and 24 hours after the fiber is removed. Antimicrobial rinses are recommended to maintain good oral hygiene. Studies indicate this treatment provides a significant reduction in pocket depth and bleeding when the tissue is touched with a probe. Improvements can be expected to be retained for six months before additional treatment is necessary.

In advanced cases the periodontist may need to perform surgery. When pockets more than 4 to 6 mm are found, it is difficult for even the dentist to remove plaque and calculus. These deep pockets invite infection and bone destruction, if they are allowed to remain untreated. *Flap surgery* is performed when pockets are deep and bone has been destroyed. This will allow the dentist to gain access to the roots of the teeth so calculus, plaque, and diseased tissue can be removed. This technique involves lifting the gum away and then suturing (stitching) it back into place or into a new position that will be easier to clean. *Osseous (bone) surgery* is sometimes performed in conjunction with flap surgery. This surgery involves reshaping some of the bone around the tooth. In certain cases, a bone graft might be performed to replace lost bone.

Splints are used to stabilize loose teeth temporarily if it is necessary after periodontal therapy.

The number of sessions and cost of periodontal treatment vary with the nature of the problem. If you should require periodontal surgery, discuss the type of surgery and the reason for your dentist's particular approach. He may suggest a hemisection, root amputation, bicuspidization (all discussed in the Endodontics chapter), or any number of other approaches. A discussion of all the possibilities is beyond the scope of this book. When in doubt, do not hesitate to get a second opinion on the proposed treatment and another estimate of the cost.

Most of these periodontal procedures require the use of pain medications; however, they are usually not needed beyond a few days. The success rate varies with the extent and nature of the problem; and thus, this should be discussed prior to beginning treatment.

THE QUIET DISEASE—DON'T WAIT UNTIL IT HURTS

"Why should I waste my money on going to the dentist when my teeth feel fine? Are checkups really necessary when your teeth are not bothering you?"

These are questions that dental professionals hear all too often. Your teeth are intended to last a lifetime, but it is going to take proper home and professional care to achieve this goal. This means you are going to have to brush thoroughly each day (after breakfast and just before bedtime), clean between the teeth with floss and/or an irrigator, and have regular professional cleanings to avoid periodontal disease. Good oral hygiene is essential to help keep periodontal disease from becoming more serious or recurring. Advanced periodontal disease is the leading cause of tooth loss in adults, but this can be prevented. Having sound teeth without sound supporting gingival tissue or bone tissue is analogous to having a soundly built house placed on a faulty foundation. The most insidious aspect of periodontal disease is that it is usually painless, and can develop either slowly or quite rapidly. Periodontal disease can get out of control quite easily if you do not have dental checkups at regular intervals. Only your dentist is able to recognize periodontal disease in its early stages. Patients are not easily able to identify early signs of periodontitis, so they are not aware they have it until their gums and bone have been so seriously damaged that tooth loss is usually inevitable. If finances are a consideration, it is considerably less expensive to treat periodontitis in its early stages. Advanced stages usually require surgery, and many times extensive restoration of the teeth and bone support.

You can find a good periodontist for yourself using the same considerations that were discussed in locating the right general dentist. Usually, if you are seeing a general dentist and you need to see a periodontist, he will suggest the name of one to you. It is important for the general dentist and the specialist to work well together, since there needs to be a compatability of philosophy.

HALITOSIS (BAD BREATH)

Bad breath is a problem that all of us experience at one time or another. For some people, however, it is a chronic problem that is so severe it is socially embarrassing and psychologically debilitating. It seems that no matter how often they brush, floss, and rinse with perfumed, alcohol-based mouth rinses they only get temporary relief.

It has been estimated that 40 percent of the population has chronic halitosis. Studies have shown that 80 percent of the time the cause of bad breath originates in the mouth, and the remainder of the time it is from other causes. In a recent ADA/Colgate Oral Health Trend Survey 63 percent of the dentists reported poor oral hygiene was the most common cause of bad breath, and 21 percent felt periodontal disease was the second most common cause of the problem. The trend indicated more men than women are treated for the problem. The survey indicated 51 percent of the dentists felt the most effective treatment for halitosis was periodic dental cleanings and oral hygiene instruction.

Some dentists feel that dead cells and bacteria in the mouth putrefy, forming volatile sulfur gases, and it is these gases that cause halitosis. They feel the spaces between and around the teeth, gums, and especially the tongue are areas where this debris is trapped. Keeping the tongue clean by brushing seems to be a very important factor in eliminating bad breath.

If you are experiencing bad breath, it is important to see a dentist for a thorough dental examination, tooth cleaning, and home care instruction. He should take a thorough medical and dental history. If you have any periodontal problems they should be treated by either the general dentist or a periodontist. Since systemic problems can contribute to bad breath, the patient should be questioned about existing oral cancers, diabetes, and liver or kidney disorders. Medical problems that involve the sinuses, tonsils and adenoids, and certain prescription medications (particularly those that cause drying of the mouth) can also be the cause of halitosis. Contrary to popular belief, many dentists feel gastrointestinal problems are not related to chronic halitosis.

The October 1995 issue of *Dentistry Today* states there are toothpastes that contain various essential oils that reduce odors. For example, oxidants such as peroxides neutralize the more noxious odors. One popular toothpaste on the market today uses chlorine dioxide, perhaps the most powerful oxidant available today.

Studies indicate there are a group of patients who just cannot seem to eliminate their halitosis with conventional treatment. Due to the increasing demand for a solution to this problem there are a number of centers across the United States that focus on the treatment of halitosis. These facilities incorporate nonsurgical periodontics with the use of home care products that neutralize the bacteria that cause bad breath. Consult your Yellow Pages for the name of a center close to you.

9

Prosthodontics

Prosthodontics entails the restoration of significant tooth structure or total replacement of a tooth or teeth. Fixed prosthetic devices in dentistry include gold *crowns* to restore a tooth that has lost gross tooth structure and dental *bridges* to replace a missing tooth or teeth. Removable prosthodontic devices that replace some or all of the teeth in an upper or lower dental arch are known as a *partial* or *full dentures*. Each of these is discussed in detail below.

If you suffer either extensive tooth or ridge loss, or if you have unusual tooth relationships, you may need a prosthodontist to correct the problem. A prosthodontist is a specialist who has had two years of additional training beyond dental school in an ADA-approved training program. His training prepares him to handle complex prosthodontic cases beyond the scope of that done by a general dentist.

For instance, if you need a full denture and you have no *dental ridge* (the bony arch that supports the roots of the teeth in the mouth) to fit the denture upon then you would probably be better served by a prosthodontist. Other examples would be if you need either a long-span bridge to replace and/or restore several adjacent teeth or extensive full-mouth reconstruction because you have so many teeth decayed or missing. Difficult cases such as these are better handled by a prosthodontist.

Prosthodontics (both fixed and removable) is done by both general dentists and specialists. Fixed prosthodontics, which includes crowns and bridges, can be removed by only a dentist. Removable prosthodontics, which includes partial and full dentures, can be removed by the patient on a regular daily basis to be cleaned. The decision about whether you should see a prosthodontist or have your treatment performed by a general dentist should be determined on an individual basis. You and your general dentist can discuss the matter, or you can make an appointment yourself to see a prosthodontist. A referral is not necessary from your general dentist. Check with the local dental society or look in your Yellow Pages in the dental specialist section under "prosthodontist" if you need one.

Human jaws were created to accommodate 32 teeth, and when these teeth are all present and healthy they work together in a very marvelous, complex, and efficient manner. A full complement of adjacent teeth in the upper and lower jaws is called a *dental arch*. The teeth in the dental arch *occlude* (bite together) when they are in normal bite position. Your mouth has two dental arches: the *maxillary* (upper arch) and the *mandibular* (lower arch). Proper functional chewing is accomplished when a full complement of teeth are correctly positioned in their opposing arches. But problems arise when all the teeth are not correctly positioned or when one or more of them is missing. This is called *malocclusion*.

Removing a tooth from the dental arch without replacing it causes stresses on the remaining teeth because the biting forces are unevenly distributed during chewing. The strength of the dental arch is lost because the remaining teeth have a tendency to shift into positions that fill in the gap. This causes the proper *contact* (space) between the teeth to be lost.

The amount of contact you have between your teeth is very important. Teeth should rest close enough to one another to cause dental floss to meet some resistance but still pass between the teeth. Too tight a contact does not allow proper cleaning or flossing between teeth. Too loose a contact allows ready accumulation of food between the teeth, resulting in *periodontitis* (tissue inflammation) and/or dental caries.

Teeth can *super-erupt* if an opposing tooth is positioned such that it has no antagonist. In these cases, the tooth from the opposing dental arch frequently erupts until it has something to oppose. Many times the contacts in this area are loose, resulting in an increased incidence of periodontitis and/or dental caries.

Now let us discuss, in more detail, fixed and removable prosthodontics.

FIXED PROSTHODONTICS

The ideal replacement for a missing tooth or excessive loss of tooth structure is some type of fixed prosthodontics. It is important to replace missing teeth to maintain the natural shape of your face and to have adequate support for your lips and cheeks. When back teeth are lost it can cause your mouth to sink and your face to look older. More importantly, your dental health suffers when teeth are not replaced because the adjacent teeth will shift toward the empty space or the teeth in the opposite jaw usually move up or down toward the space. This not only causes stress on the tissues and remaining teeth in your mouth, but it also increases the risk of gum disease. Teeth that have shifted are difficult to clean, making them more likely candidates for decay. This can result in losing even more teeth. Missing teeth also affect the way you chew and speak. When you chew on only one side it can cause stress to your mouth. Your teeth also contribute to your ability to speak properly because they help you make the many sounds needed in speech.

Fixed prosthetic devices include: a crown, which replaces a tooth that has extensively destroyed tooth structure; or a bridge, which is a tooth-replacing prosthesis having one or more crowns that serve as an *abutment* to anchor the bridge to existing teeth when it is cemented into place. An *abutment* on a bridge is the anchor (or support) tooth on either side of the space where a tooth is missing. A bridge also includes a *pontic* (the unit of the bridge that is the replacement for the missing tooth). Each tooth and each pontic in the bridge is considered a *unit*.

Crowns and bridges are custom-made restorations that are fabricated from either alloys (gold or nonprecious metals) or porcelain. There are several choices of crowns to consider. Crown restorations can be composed of gold, porcelain, porcelain fused to metal (PFM), or even plastic. Since very few crowns are composed of plastics, this discussion will be limited to the first three options.

Crowns made of alloys are not esthetic because they are not the color of natural teeth. However, where esthetics is not necessarily a consideration, as in the instance of posterior (back) teeth, these crowns are an excellent restoration when done properly. It is very common to use porcelain bonded to a metal shell because it is both esthetic and strong. Bridges can be made of the same materials as single-unit crowns. Your choice of an alloy or a type of porcelain ceramic material will thus depend on financial and esthetic considerations.

Fixed prosthetic devices are cemented by the dentist over existing tooth structure, and thus cannot be removed by the patient. This differs from removable prosthetic devices in that those are removed by the patient on a regular basis for cleaning.

Before a fixed prosthetic device can be placed, either as a single unit or as part of a bridge, the tooth (or teeth) must be reduced in size. The dentist refers to this procedure as tooth "reduction" or tooth "preparation."

The tooth must be reduced in size for two reasons. First, tooth reduction of the *occlusal* (chewing) surface is necessary because an allowance has to be made for the width of the material used in the crown.

Teeth are so sensitive on biting down that objects the thickness of a human hair can be felt between the teeth. If the occlusal surface of the tooth to be crowned was not reduced, whenever you chewed, you would prematurely bite down on the crowned tooth before you bit on any other teeth. This not only would be annoying, but would also make the tooth sore. In short, you could not chew!

Second, the tooth must be reduced on all surfaces that will be covered to allow room for the proper contour of the tooth. This reduction allows space so that the tooth can be both esthetic-looking and have proper contacts (space between the teeth). Tooth contour is important to maintain good periodontal health.

Fixed prosthestic devices do not come in sizes as do shoes, so they must be custom-made to fit properly. Usually the patient needs to see the dentist for two visits. On the first visit the dentist will prepare the tooth (or teeth), take an impression, get a correct bite relationship, and get a correct shade for the replacement teeth (if porcelain is to be used).

When taking an impression, the dentist will use a tray that fits the contour of your dental arch. A sticky impression material is placed into the tray to take an impression of both the prepared tooth and adjacent teeth. After this sticky impression material sets to a non-sticky elastic consistency, it is removed from your mouth. The impression is filled with a plasterlike material. When the plasterlike material sets, this provides a model (duplicate) of your teeth to be used to create the proper dimensions for the future crown. The only dimension lacking is the opposing occlusion for the new crown. This is obtained by taking another impression of the opposing teeth, which is also poured up in a plasterlike material.

Proper occlusion (bite) is as important as proper fit, contour, and contacts with adjacent teeth. An articulator is used to mount the models in proper occlusion. An articulator is a mechanical hingelike device that simulates the jaw's biting actions.

The dentist or his assistant will usually make a "temporary" crown from acrylic resins to cover each prepared tooth while the permanent crown or bridge is being made. If the shape or length of your tooth is being changed for cosmetic reasons, the temporary crowns will allow you time to get used to this change. This gives you time to make changes before the permanent crown or bridge is made.

Most dentists do not make crowns or bridges for their patients. This is the function of a dental technician working in a dental laboratory.

When the final fixed prosthetic device is ready at the lab, you will need to see your dentist for a second visit so he can seat it in place and make any necessary adjustments.

Crowns and bridges must be kept very, very clean. The ultimate success or failure of fixed prosthetic devices depends on their foundation.

It is especially important to keep plaque removed from the area where the gum meets the tooth because it can cause tooth decay or gum disease. Be sure to clean the areas under, around, and between a bridge and your natural teeth. Dental floss threaders and interdental cleaners (specially shaped brushes as well as rubber, plastic, or wooden items) can help you reach these areas. You should avoid chewing hard foods and ice to help prevent damage to your esthetic crowns.

Crowns

A crown is a restoration that covers a tooth to restore its original shape and size. It strengthens and improves the appearance of the tooth. Crowns are usually suggested as a replacement for one of the following reasons:

1. to support a tooth that is very severely destroyed by dental caries or trauma
2. to restore a tooth that has had root canal therapy
3. to attach a bridge
4. to restore fractured teeth
5. to cover badly shaped or discolored teeth

For the restoration of front teeth, most people want a natural look. They do not want the "metal look" every time they laugh or yawn. Thus, the choice is either porcelain or PFM crowns because they are tooth-colored. However, these esthetic crowns cost more than the alloy crown (see the chapter on dental fees).

There are some problems with esthetic crowns. Porcelain is not as durable as alloy, so sometimes these crowns fracture and leave behind exposed dentin. The PFM crowns can fracture off their porcelain, leaving behind an uncovered thimble of alloy.

No matter what material is used in the restoring crown, the retention of it depends on how much tooth structure the crown rests upon. On occasion, the underlying preparation must be built up to gain adequate retention.

For ideal strength and retention the crown must be placed on at least 2 mm of good marginal tooth structure. A technique called *crown lengthening* can sometimes "lengthen" the tooth, if the tooth does not have an adequate amount of tooth structure. This procedure is done prior to preparing the tooth for the crown to be sure adequate length can be accomplished.

Bridges

Bridges are composed of a series of crowns and one or more pontics soldered together to form a single unit to replace the space where one or more teeth have been lost. Crowns placed on teeth located at either side of the missing teeth comprise the *abutments* (the stabilizing supports for a bridge). The replacement teeth attached to the abutments are called *pontics*. Pontics are artificial teeth used to fill the space left by missing teeth. They are usually soldered to the crowns of the abutment teeth to form a solid unit (the bridge). Or pontics can be attached to the crown of an abutment tooth on only one side. This latter example is called a *cantilever bridge*. Today, many authorities feel that the only successful cantilever bridges are those limited to the anterior (front) teeth. This is because chewing on the anterior teeth produces minimal forces. This is an important concept to remember because a cantilever bridge, as its name implies, has lever action. A lever provides a great mechanical advantage in moving objects. This same lever action can occur in a cantilever bridge. Therefore, it is important for the cantilever bridge to be constructed with adequate support for the stresses it must withstand. Otherwise, the bone support of the abutment tooth could be destroyed and the bridge would fail.

How many abutments are necessary to support the necessary pontics properly? A dental bridge is not unlike a bridge that spans an expanse of water or a deep natural depression in the earth's terrain. Engineers in charge of constructing a bridge across a natural expanse must consider the length of the bridge, the amount of weight or stress the bridge must be able to withstand, and the type of materials and supports that are necessary to accommodate the stresses. Dentists ask themselves these same questions when designing a bridge for you.

Engineers know one end of a bridge cannot be anchored in quicksand and be expected to support any significant load. Neither can a dental bridge be expected to support a load when it is anchored on one end to a tooth that has lost considerable bony support because of periodontal disease. Bridges to replace one missing tooth do not need to be supported by teeth with as much root and bone support as a bridge to replace multiple missing teeth would need. In this section devoted to fixed prosthodontics, it is impossible to give more than very generalized rules for constructing sound bridges. Patients must realize that for every rule there are exceptions because of individual needs or constraints.

Three unit bridges are perhaps the most popular. These bridges have two abutments and one pontic. In other words, they are used to replace a single missing tooth. Three unit bridges are ideal because they present maximum bridge strength. In general, there should be at least one abutment for every pontic in sound bridge design.

Another type of bridge available is the *Maryland bridge*. The easiest way to describe a Maryland bridge is to visualize a pontic seated in place with a wire mesh coming out from both its sides. It is not necessary to prepare the teeth and place crowns because the wire mesh is attached to each abutment tooth by a special procedure called *bonding*. The cost is less than the conventional bridges discussed above because the abutment teeth do not have to be reduced for crowns, as with conventional bridges. The biggest disadvantage of the Maryland bridge is that the acid etch material may break away from the abutment tooth and must be reattached by your dentist. This type of bridge is commonly used for anterior tooth replacement. Often two adjacent teeth on each side of the missing tooth (teeth) are incorporated into the bridge to give it extra strength.

In recent years dentists have begun supporting bridges with implants. This has enabled prosthetic devices that otherwise would not be possible to be fabricated.

Fixed bridges are not always possible because of the extent of the space or lack of sound abutments. Here is where the removable tooth replacements are a good option to consider.

REMOVABLE PROSTHODONTICS

Dentures have been around for more than 2,000 years. Today, they are of better quality and are more comfortable than in previous generations. As the name implies, a removable prosthodontic appliance can be taken out of and put back into the mouth. *Full dentures* replace all the teeth in either the upper (*maxillary*) or lower (*mandibular*) dental arch, or both. Here the only "anchor" for the denture is the *dental ridge* itself. *Partial dentures* replace missing teeth that cannot be replaced with a bridge either because of the large number of teeth missing or the location of the missing teeth. A partial denture, which is basically a part of a "full" denture, is both tooth and tissue supported. More specifically, key remaining teeth and the dental ridge in the arch are both incorporated to support the appliance so that the biting forces are distributed among the remaining teeth and tissue.

According to a study at University of Pennsylvania approximately 20 percent (one adult member in about one-half of all households) of the population in the United States wears either full or partial dentures. Of this group, about 50 percent are under 65 years old.

Both general dentists and prosthodontists make dentures (full or partial). If you lack adequate ridge support for the denture base to rest upon, have difficulty wearing your present denture, or have some other unique denture-related problem, you should probably consult a prosthodontist rather than a general dentist. His special training has given him a better insight on how to treat difficult cases properly.

Teeth should not be saved because your dentist wants you to save them. This decision should be made by you because you are aware of the importance of maintaining your teeth. In particular, you should be aware that no prosthesis exists that acts as an adequate substitute for a natural tooth. That makes your natural teeth very valuable to you.

The usual procedure after the decision has been made to have dentures is as follows:

1. Impression(s) of the existing teeth and ridges are taken
2. A model (replica of the existing teeth and ridge) is constructed by filling the final impressions with a plasterlike material that sets to a hard consistency
3. A jaw relationship (the correct bite) of the patient's existing upper and lower teeth and/or ridge is determined
4. The models are then placed in a device that securely holds them in the proper biting relationship just determined
5. The same teeth that will be extracted are removed from the models (for immediate dentures only)
6. The models are sent to the lab with instructions for the denture base to be made in wax using the same teeth that will be used in the completed denture
7. The patient is allowed to try on the "wax" denture to check the looks and fit
8. The wax denture is sent to the lab and the final denture is constructed

If you have no existing teeth or perhaps an existing denture, it is usually a routine matter to have a new denture constructed and placed. But if you have teeth that must be extracted and replaced with a denture, there are at least two ways this can be accomplished.

First, the obvious way to replace natural teeth with dentures is to extract the teeth, let the extraction sites heal, then finally have the denture constructed to fit the healed ridges. The only problem with this treatment plan is the delay until the tissue is healed enough for the denture to be made. Most people do not want to be seen in public without their teeth.

Immediate dentures are another option to consider when having dentures made. With this technique, the denture is constructed ahead of time and then placed in the mouth immediately after the teeth are extracted. Therefore the patient is never without his teeth. More about this technique in the upcoming section on immediate dentures.

Dentures: Why You Don't Want Them

Most people do not realize the problems that arise after dentures are placed. How would you like to have an artificial leg rather than your natural leg? I feel on very safe ground in assuming that you would emphatically answer: "Definitely not!"

Replacing your natural teeth with either a full or partial denture is about as desirable as having an artificial leg. Dentures allow you to chew; an artificial leg allows you to walk. The problem in both instances is the performance quality of the artificial replacement in comparison to what nature originally provided. Quite simply, the artificial replacement will never function as well as your natural teeth.

Dentures are not maintenance free; they need adjustments. It is not that the dentures change; it is the tissues under the dentures that change. A denture adjustment is necessary when the denture material must be removed from the denture to relieve pressure at pressure spots that occur when bone and tissue shrink.

Since tissue shrinks as it heals, dentures that are placed immediately after the teeth are extracted need to be relined as soon as the tissue has healed. All dentures need relining periodically to adjust for normal tissue changes. So a denture is not a one-shot cure. It is very important to see your dentist once a year so the tissue under the denture can be monitored.

With this overview, let me offer a word of caution. Your dentist may offer you options on the types of tooth replacements possible in your case. Offering you treatment options is part of your dentist's obligation. This is where you need to become a wise, informed dental consumer so you can discuss with him the best decision for your situation.

As a general rule of thumb, fixed prosthodontics (crowns and bridges) are more expensive than removable prosthodontics (full or partial dentures). However, fixed prosthodontics are usually a more desirable replacement. Dentures also vary in cost depending on the type of teeth, the material used to make the denture base, and the number of steps followed to construct the prosthetic device. If you find a place that claims to be able to make your denture in one day for much less than the fee being charged in the area by most other dentists, you will probably get exactly what you pay for. Let the buyer beware! There are no bargains in health care!

Immediate Dentures

The name *immediate dentures* sounds like something produced by a fast-food version of a dental office. However, "immediate" in this context means that the denture is placed immediately after the dentist or the oral and maxillofacial surgeon extracts the teeth.

Here is a typical example of what happens in preparation for an immediate denture. The first phase is the removal of all the teeth posterior to (behind) the cuspid teeth. These ridges are then allowed to heal and act as a stable base for the future denture. After the healing has occurred, the denture is constructed as previously described in the Removable Prosthodontics section. Then, the natural teeth are extracted and the dentures are immediately placed in the mouth. This keeps the patient from having to be without his or her anterior (front) teeth at any time.

There are many advantages to immediate dentures, besides the immediate esthetic considerations. They protect the sensitive extraction sites, help control bleeding from the tooth sockets, and protect the surgical area by covering it, thus keeping food and debris out of the extraction sockets.

An additional advantage that you might consider worth the extra expense of the immediate denture is that your dentist knows how your "natural" teeth appeared. Thus, he is likely to be able to construct a denture that more closely resembles your natural teeth. This makes the transition easier when you see your friends and family because your appearance is minimally changed. The other option is that it is possible, if you want, to change your appearance with the new dentures.

Finally, an immediate denture gives the dentist a better idea of how your natural teeth were biting. He can then construct a denture that better simulates the bite you had before the extractions.

Esthetically, immediate dentures are a better way to have dentures inserted than having dentures made after going through a period of toothlessness. However, they do present more problems.

More denture adjustments are needed when immediate dentures are placed, and these dentures always need to be relined (have material placed inside the denture in the area where the denture fits against the ridge in the mouth) a short time after they are seated. The reason is that the tissue, including the bone in the area, shrinks during the healing process after the teeth are removed. The healing process lasts about six months. This shrinking causes the denture to become loose, and the fit is altered. Relining is not needed as soon for conventional dentures fitted on ridges where time has lapsed after the teeth are extracted.

Usually, the immediate dentures themselves are not any more expensive than conventional dentures. However, since immediate dentures have to be relined as soon as the ridges have healed, the reline is usually an additional charge.

Overdentures

An overdenture is a full denture that is secured to the roots of natural teeth that have had root canal therapy and crowns. Retaining the roots of your natural teeth not only helps maintain the dental ridge but also contributes to the overall stability of the prosthesis. Overdentures allow the forces of chewing to be distributed uniformly over the roots and denture-supporting soft tissues. If the retained roots are lost, the overdenture can be easily modified (converted) to a conventional denture. Even though an overdenture is more expensive than a conventional denture, the additional support that it lends is well worth the added expense.

Sometimes there are either too few teeth and/or the existing teeth have too little periodontal support to restore the dentition with either a fixed bridge or a removable partial denture. But if there are between one and four teeth within a dental ridge that are restorable and have good periodontal support, these teeth can sometimes be used to support an overdenture.

I feel that maintaining even a single root under a denture is well worth the expense since this will provide at least one area where the dental ridge is maintained. Maintaining roots on two sides of the ridge in the dental arch is even better. Most authorities agree that the optimal position and number of roots under an overdenture are two nonadjacent teeth on each side of the dental ridge. They are easy to clean, and they give better balance to the support of the overdenture. For example, it would be good to retain the cuspid and a second premolar on both sides of the dental ridge.

Dental ridges are the support (the *periodontium*) of the roots of the teeth. The presence of teeth is directly related to maintaining the presence of the dental ridges. One of the most significant problems that full denture wearers face is the loss (or *resorption*) of their supporting dental ridges, which then results in an ill-fitting denture.

An overdenture is a potential solution to the problem of ridge resorption. In an overdenture, the dentist saves the tooth root. The tooth's crown is removed and the remaining root is then contoured to resemble the shape of the existing ridge so that the denture can be placed on the ridge without interference. Chapter 1, which contains an illustration of a typical tooth, shows that the dentist cannot simply cut off a tooth's crown without exposing the root canal space. This means that root canal therapy is necessary on any tooth that is to be maintained under an overdenture.

After root canal therapy is completed the tooth is usually restored with a crown. On occasion, some dentists will use special snaplike attachments (similar to snaps on a shirt or coat) instead of a crown to attach the overdenture to the remaining roots. The snaps are fixed to the top of the remaining root and to the base of the overdenture.

Most patients need overdentures because they have not taken good care of their natural teeth. Overdenture patients must be told of the paramount importance of day-to-day care and followups with their dentist. Both the overdenture and the retained roots need to be closely monitored by a dentist because the patient will not be able to detect decay. Some dentists feel sealants should be placed on the exposed tooth roots. Daily application of fluoride to the root surfaces is also suggested. Patients must take particular care to wash the overdenture after every meal to remove any trapped food. In addition, the retained roots must also be kept very clean.

A five-year followup study of overdenture failures was done at the University of Southern California School of Dentistry. This study indicated that the retained tooth roots under the overdentures had to be extracted most frequently because of periodontal breakdown. This only emphasizes the need for keeping the retained roots and denture clean.

An overdenture is a great advantage when dentures are needed. However, an overdenture requires as much maintenance as natural teeth.

Partial Dentures

A partial denture is a removable appliance for tooth replacement that is both tooth- and tissue-supported. It is usually composed of a metal framework with the replacement teeth on an attached acrylic (plasticlike) base that rests on the dental ridge. The base is made of the same material used to construct full dentures. The metal framework of the partial denture attaches to your natural teeth with either delicate clasps that fit around the abutment teeth or devices called precision attachments. Most authorities feel precision attachments are more secure than metal clasps, and they are nearly invisible. Precision attachments generally are more expensive than metal clasps. Usually crowns are placed on the *abutment* teeth (the teeth used to secure the clasps or precision attachments) to improve the fit of the partial denture and to add extra strength to these teeth so they can support the stresses produced by chewing forces when using the partial denture. The abutment teeth must have the proper contours to attain the maximum appliance stability and retention. More specifically, the teeth must be contoured so that the appliance has retention, but can still be removed to be cleaned.

It is important that the teeth that serve as abutments (or supports) for the partial denture be sound. "Sound" means that the teeth have had root canal therapy completed, if it is necessary; that the teeth are not periodontally diseased; and that they have adequate bone support.

Generally, a partial denture is recommended for a patient who has too many missing teeth for proper support with a fixed bridge. Therefore, the missing teeth are replaced with a prosthetic appliance that will distribute the biting forces among the remaining teeth and tissue. A limited budget may be another factor for choosing a partial denture because it is usually less expensive than fixed appliances.

When the partial denture is first placed in your mouth by your dentist, he should show you how to put it in and how to take it out. Practice this several times before leaving his office. Remember that you must never use a biting force to position the appliance. If you ever force the partial denture into position, you risk bending the framework and/or possibly bending or breaking the delicate clasps.

Be careful to avoid dropping your removable appliance. This could damage the framework. Most authorities would agree that more harm can come to your removable appliance while it is out of your mouth than when it is in it. If you have problems, call your dentist immediately. *Please do not attempt to do your own adjustments.*

At first, the partial denture, like the full denture, feels bulky. No partial denture will work as well or feel as comfortable as your natural teeth. You must learn to use this artificial appliance by practicing with it when you speak and eat. The intent of the appliance is to give you better chewing function. This is similar to learning to use an artificial limb. Sore spots frequently result from areas of excessive pressure on or along the dental ridge where the partial denture rides during use.

The partial denture in professional circles is known as a "garbage collector" because food gets on and under the base, the framework, and the clasps. Lack of proper cleaning will result in caries (decay) on both abutment and other remaining teeth.

Finally, a partial denture is not a cure-all. After a period of time the partial denture will remain virtually unchanged. It is your mouth that changes. When looseness or rocking occurs, it is a sign that you should see your dentist to have your partial relined or, possibly, remade. He will usually recommend the proper time intervals between your checkups with him. It cannot be overemphasized that keeping these appointments is very important to the health of your mouth.

Denture Adhesives

Denture adhesives are products sold over the counter to help denture wearers make their denture fit more tightly on the dental ridge. These products are placed inside the denture so that when the denture is placed in the mouth it will better adhere to the shape of the dental ridge. Hence, the term "denture adhesive" is used for this material. Essentially, it is a temporary relining of the inside of the denture base with a soft material.

To have a better understanding of why denture wearers turn to adhesives, you must consider the functions of a denture. First, dentures are a replacement for missing teeth. Second, and perhaps most important, dentures function in an environment of constant movement and activity. The denture wearer's problem is to manage to keep the denture stable amid all this movement and activity. Part of the answer to denture stability may be a denture adhesive.

A new denture wearer has to relearn talking, chewing, etc. Some denture wearers want assistance to help keep their new denture in place and make them functional. Many authorities believe that it may take one to three years for a denture wearer to get accustomed to wearing and using dentures. That is a very long time. It is during this break-in period that denture adhesives are most likely to be used and/or needed. A denture adhesive can be a coping tool, providing the denture wearer a sense of control.

The ADA Seal has been given to very few denture adhesives on the market today. If you are shopping for a denture adhesive, look for this Seal to insure that the product is safe and effective, and to be sure that the manufacturer's claims are true. Patients should beware of denture pads and denture self-reliner products. These cause uneven pressure on the ridge which will almost invariably cause bone ridge loss (resorption). Even dentists have difficulty in properly relining an old denture. The consumer who tries to be an "amateur dentist" is very likely to get into trouble.

Over 250 medications used by patients (tranquilizers, diuretics, etc.) can cause dry mouth. It has been suggested that patients with dry mouths may not have enough saliva to wet the powder adhesives uniformly. This can cause sore spots because of an uneven spreading of the powdered adhesive. In these instances, it is recommended that patients use a cream or paste adhesive.

It has been documented (excluding the cases of dry mouth mentioned above) that it makes no difference whether you use cream, paste, or powder adhesive. Dr. Malcolm Brown of the University of Indiana School of Dentistry notes that marketing researchers have found that 20 percent of denture wearers are regular adhesive users.

Dentures do not last forever. Since tissues change, you do need regular periodic checkups on your denture by your dentist. Do not try to mask over or live with a problem denture. Adhesives are only meant to be used with properly fitting dentures.

Dentures . . . Wearing and Caring

The wearing of and caring for dentures (whether they are immediate dentures, full dentures, or partial dentures) go together like a hand and a glove. You cannot properly wear a denture without properly caring for it.

The wearing of a new denture is a unique experience. One problem you may have is that it takes time for the muscles of your cheeks and lips to adjust to the denture if you are a first time denture wearer. If you have had several back teeth missing prior to getting your new denture, you probably had a "sunken in" look. A denture will aid in restoring the facial image you had prior to any extractions.

They key to wearing any denture is attitude. A positive attitude is paramount to wearing any prosthesis successfully, whether it is a replacement for an arm, leg, or your teeth. You must develop realistic expectations and realize that nothing will ever function as well as what you have lost.

The initial problems you can expect with your new denture include a bulky and loose feeling, excessive saliva flow, a feeling that the tongue does not have adequate room, and difficulty in both eating and speaking. You will adjust to these problems if you are patient and maintain a good attitude.

You will learn to control the denture, but this will take time. Think of wearing dentures as an athletic feat, for which you need a coach. The coach is your dentist.

Here are a few hints you might consider in learning to eat correctly: start by eating soft foods, cut your food into small pieces, chew your food on both sides of your back teeth at the same time to prevent the dentures from tipping, and use caution in eating foods that are hot or have bones. Dentures cover the dental ridge so it is hard to sense heat or foods that could possibly choke you (bones or toothpicks). Be careful of sticky foods, especially at first.

Practice speaking with the denture by reading aloud. It will take practice to pronounce certain words. If your dentures have a tendency to "click together" while you are speaking, try speaking more slowly. If speaking problems persist bring it to the attention of your dentist. He may need to make some adjustments for you.

Most dentists prefer their patients not to wear their dentures at night to allow the tissue time to rest. Go on the advice of your dentist for your particular needs. If you do take your dentures out remember they will warp if they are allowed to dry out or if they are exposed to hot water. Most dentists recommend they be kept in a denture cleanser soaking solution when they are not in your mouth.

There are some general guidelines to keep in mind regarding the care of your denture. Always remember they are very delicate and may break if dropped. When handling them it is best to stand over a folded towel or a basin of water. Like natural teeth, dentures must be brushed with a denture cleanser in the morning, after meals, and before going to bed to remove food deposits and plaque. This will not only keep your mouth fresh and healthy, but it will also help prevent the denture from becoming permanently stained. It is best to use a brush designed for dentures, but a regular toothbrush with soft bristles can be used. You can clean your denture with hand soap, mild dishwashing liquid, or denture cleanser recommended by your dentist. Never use powdered household cleansers because they are too abrasive. The best approach is to look for the Seal of Acceptance of the ADA on products you use, as discussed in chapter 1. Ultrasonic cleaners can also be used, but they are not a substitute for daily brushing. Don't forget to also brush your palate, tongue, and gingiva daily with a soft bristled brush. Pets and children are a potential source of damage to your denture, so keep it out of their reach.

Most dentists do not recommend that denture adhesives be used for a prolonged period of time. If your denture is loose you need to see your dentist to avoid having problems with tissue irritation. Adjustments are a normal part of denture wear, and they should be taken care of in a timely manner. An unattended denture sore could contribute to the development of oral cancer.

Never try to fix your own denture. Many times this results in making it necessary to make new dentures because your home handiwork has made them irreparable and unable to be worn. If your tooth breaks, cracks, chips, or becomes loose or falls out your dentist can often repair it on the same day. A denture that does not fit properly can cause tissue irritation and sores.

Long-term wear and care on your denture means getting at least an annual checkup. Over a period of time, your denture will need to be relined, remade, or *rebased* due to normal wear. Rebasing a denture involves making a new denture base that incorporates the existing denture teeth. As a person ages, his mouth naturally changes. Bone and gum ridges shrink, causing the bite to change and the dentures to fit loosely. Since this makes chewing difficult and many times causes tissue irritation, it is important to see your dentist to have your denture and mouth evaluated.

10

Public Health Dentistry

A public health dental specialist is a dentist who has had at least two years of training beyond dental school in an ADA-accredited program. The number of public health dentists is small, and their primary function is usually not direct patient care. They primarily serve as dental health planners, advisers, and educators. They plan and advise state and federal governments on issues that directly influence the quality and the quantity of dental care you receive as a dental consumer. For instance, they study and advise on such issues as smokeless (chewing) tobacco, measures to avoid transmission of communicable diseases, and taxation of health benefits. At the present time, they are involved in the nationwide program called Oral Health 2000. Their goal is to involve 75 percent of all dentists in the United States in organized intervention plans for people who either smoke or use smokeless tobacco. They want dentists to begin providing tobacco-cessation programs by offering assistance through counseling, nicotine patches or gum, and more thorough oral health care. Effective January 1, 1995, a special ADA code (01320) has been created for the dentist to use to bill insurance companies for "Tobacco Counseling for the Control and Prevention of Oral Disease." Another goal of the Oral Health 2000 project is for 50 percent of all children to have sealants placed on their teeth.

The U.S. Public Health Service (PHS) is under the control of the Department of Health and Human Services. It is the principal health agency of the federal government. Since its creation in 1798, the Public Health Service has grown to include eight agencies. They are the Agency for Health Care Policy and Research, the Agency for Toxic Substances and Disease Registry; the Alcohol, Drug Abuse and Mental Health Administration, the Centers for Disease Control; the Food and Drug Administration; Health Resources and Services Administration; Indian Health Service; and National Institute of Health. The National Institute of Dental Research (NIDR) is under the National Institute of Health. It is at this level that dental research and planning is done. There are 16 NIDR centers in the United States. These centers can be divided into two categories: specialized centers and basic centers. Eleven specialized NIDR centers deal primarily with dental caries and periodontal disease research. Five NIDR basic centers work on a multitude of dentally related issues.

NIDR researchers include dental specialists and other scientists (many are not dentists), such as physiologists, anatomists, and biochemists. Their research is done under research grants and contracts from the federal government and private agencies.

The public health dental specialists are included on the committees that decide where and how the research monies should be used. They are included because they are experts in knowing where the dental health problems lie and which ones should be given priority.

Most of the NIDR centers are associated with dental schools. This is where advising, providing services, and educating overlap. Public health issues are taught as part of every dental school curriculum.

The dentists who work for the Public Health Service and serve as primary care providers are not public health specialists. They are general dentists who have a salaried position. They provide direct care to patients who are eligible for public health dental benefits. This would include providing dental services to American Indians and Alaska natives, federal prisoners, and Coast Guard personnel.

The original PHS hospitals that were staffed by PHS dentists were created to treat merchant seamen. Most of these have since been closed. PHS hospitals still exist, but the majority are now for treatment of American Indians and Alaska natives.

As dental care providers, the PHS dentists do not charge the patients they treat for their services. Federal funding is used to operate PHS hospitals. The PHS is not meant to be a substitute for private practice. Therefore, these dentists provide only basic care, with primary emphasis on prevention. Basic care usually involves fillings and extractions. Maintenance and/or prevention of dental disease involves brushing, flossing, regular checkups, and so on.

PART III

Trends, Fears, and Issues in Dentistry

11

Issues in Dentistry

entistry is not what it used to be, and it probably will never return to its former status. Managed dental care is a major issue that is on the minds of everyone involved. It has created a huge amount of paperwork and ethical concerns for the participating dentists, and many patients have become disillusioned with the strict guidelines and limited coverage of the plans. Due to the financial burden the plans place on the participating dentists, there are now fewer dentists willing to participate in the plans, making it even more difficult for patients to receive treatment. More on this issue will be discussed in the chapter on dental insurance.

Additionally, overtures are being made by some dental technicians, calling themselves *denturists*, to be allowed to provide direct care to patients who need dentures. They argue the cost will be less expensive to patients. Again, the question is raised whether quality or quantity of service is the most important objective.

Other issues dentistry is facing include providing care for the elderly. Along with the new technology of today a large group of baby boomers are approaching their later years. Unlike their parents, they have retained most of their teeth, which has created a whole new group of concerns for dentists who are treating them. Fluoride is still being debated by some consumer groups, even though its introduction into the city water supplies has almost eliminated dental caries. The use of sedation (intravenous, oral, and nitrous oxide/oxygen) in the office is still a controversial issue. Many states have addressed some concerns related to this matter, but the issue is far from settled.

Dealing with handicapped and fearful dental patients who have neglected their teeth presents unique problems. Better ways of handling this special group of patients have been introduced. The use of lasers in dentistry has created quite a stir. Research is still under way to discover even more areas where this new technology can be used in dentistry.

Tobacco use cessation and oral health is now being addressed by a huge government project called Oral Health 2000. Their goal is to encourage dentists to actively intervene to decrease by 75 percent the use of tobacco by the year 2000.

And finally, with the introduction of the new guidelines for health professionals by the Occupational Health and Safety Administration (OSHA) and the CDC there has been a dramatic increase in the occurence of latex allergies. The above are only a few of the current dental issues. Each will be discussed in the following sections.

DENTURISTS AND DENTURISM

A non-dentist who takes impressions and fabricates a patient's full or partial denture from start to finish, including adjusting, relining, etc. is called a denturist. Denturists work without the supervision of a dentist. The first denturists in the United States were and still are dental laboratory technicians. Most of these individuals learn their trade by on-the-job training, although some do attend formal training courses that last from six months to two years.

Denturism has been legal in Canada for over 25 years, and schools for denturism have existed there for many years. It is estimated that denturists provide over half of the dentures for Canadians. However, requirements for licensure vary greatly from province to province. Their national organization is called the National Denturists Association (NDA). Denturists in the United States have formed an organized group for purposes of gaining licensure under the name Citizens for Affordable Dental Care. Their platform is based on freedom of choice, price, and free enterprise. Legislation to legalize denturism in the United States has, at this writing, been passed in Arizona, Colorado, Idaho, Maine, Montana, Oregon, and Washington. Initiative proposals were started in 32 other states, but fell short.

There is a tremendous amount of controversy in this country surrounding denturism. In addition to allowing denturists to make and fit complete or partial dentures, the proposals call for educational requirements for those that want to become denturists in the future. However, at this writing there are no schools in place to train denturists in the United States. Probably the most controversial aspect of some proposals is a grandfather clause that allows anyone currently practicing denturism to become licensed without meeting any specific educational requirements. Many opponents to denturism feel it is a bad public policy to allow illegal activity to be a prerequisite for licensure.

In addition, opponents feel that providing dentures and partials is a health care service, not a matter of selling a product. They remind the public that before a denture or partial is made it is very important for overall oral health to be evaluated, and denturists simply do not have the training to conduct a proper evaluation. Many dentists have come forth to give testimonials about patients who have experienced serious problems at the hands of denturists. Denturists do not have the training to be able to take X rays, restore or extract teeth, perform periodontal treatment, determine jaw relationships, or recognize the origin of oral lesions such as cancer or hyperplasia. Therefore, opponents question how they can make partial or full dentures. Many consumers remain unclear on the differences between dentists and denturists. As I have already pointed out, there is a definite difference in the training and background of a dentist and a denturist. Patients need to be concerned about the quality of the treatment they are receiving. Both full and partial denture patients need the same specialized care from well-trained people as patients with any other dental problem.

A dental consumer who is considering using a denturist should consider certain facts and issues carefully. I have already pointed out in the chapter on prosthodontics the steps necessary to make a denture (full or partial), the options to consider, and the problems to be expected with these appliances. With this information at hand, I do not see how an informed consumer could choose a denturist when it comes to their dental care. There are serious consequences if these issues are not addressed before an appliance is made, not to mention the necessary followup care that is needed. There is certainly more to this issue than insuring public access to inexpensive dentures.

There are already access programs in place in this country that enable patients in the lower socioeconomic group to obtain dentures on a fee scale based on their income (or lack of income). These access programs are run and sponsored by trained, licensed dentists.

The *Seattle Times* identified the issue quite well in an editorial when they commented that the legislation for denturism was "a misguided and unnecessary proposal foisted upon voters by a tiny special-interest group that virtually bought a spot on the ballot."

DENTISTRY FOR THE ELDERLY

The elderly population has been subdivided by authorities into the following categories: 1) ages 65–74 are considered to be "young" elderly, and they are usually healthy and active, 2) ages 75–84 are considered to be "mid-old" and vary from being healthy and active to those with an array of chronic diseases, 3) age 85 and older are considered "oldest old" and are usually more frail physically.

The U.S. Census Bureau has projected that by the year 2000 approximately 13 percent (34.9 million) of the population in the U.S. will be 65 years old or older, and by the year 2030 this group will include 21.8 percent (67.4 million) of the population. In 1960 fewer than 45 percent of this population retained some or all of their natural teeth, but today the figure has grown to 60 percent. A recent study at the University of North Carolina at Chapel Hill indicated elderly blacks are almost twice as likely as elderly whites to lose their teeth. Periodontal disease is the major cause of tooth loss in adults today.

Periodontal Disease

The elderly of today consider good oral health an integral part of attaining an overall improved quality of life, so we will likely see an increased demand for periodontal treatment in this age group. Treating older patients represents an opportunity and a challenge to periodontists because this segment of the population is retaining their natural teeth, and thus they are at greater risk for periodontal disease. A recent clinical study funded by the National Institute of Aging on a group of patients ages 70–96 revealed this group has a substantially higher incidence of periodontal disease than previously estimated. Another study of patients in this age group concluded that 16 percent of the white subjects had severe periodontal disease when compared to 46 percent of the black patients.

Most gum disease is caused by bacteria that create toxins that irritate the gums, and eventually causes the gums to detach from the teeth. If left untreated, the supporting bone dissolves and the teeth become loose and finally fall out. Other conditions that increase the severity of periodontal disease are ill-fitting dentures or bridges, poor diets and/or oral hygiene, some medical diseases, and even some medications. There are more than 300 compounds in medications today that can cause an increase in the incidence of periodontitis. The medications that cause xerostomia (dry mouth) include: immunosuppressants, calcium-channel blockers, nonsteroidal anti-inflammatory agents, and antimicrobials. Environmental factors such as stress, smoking, and systemic diseases can also affect the elderly's risk factor to periodontal disease. It was recently reported that people being medicated with beta blockers, diuretics, anticholinergics, synthroid, and allopurinol had a significant decrease in calculus (compared to nonmedicated counterparts), but had a high quantity of plaque. Many elderly people complain their teeth seem darker, but the fact is they have a buildup of plaque and the teeth just seem to look darker.

Symptoms of periodontal disease include bleeding and tender gums, constant bad breath, receding gums, and loose teeth. Proper home care and regular checkups by your dentist can insure early intervention and treatment of this disease. Your teeth can last a lifetime!

Dry Mouth

Dr. Ronald Ettinger at the University of Iowa Geriatric Dental Program reports, "These elderly patients also tend to have dental problems complicated by chronic diseases and multiple drug therapies." For instance, many medications taken by elderly contribute to burning sensations in the mouth, difficulty in speaking and/or swallowing, and dry mouth (which can cause tooth decay). Saliva is needed to lubricate the mouth, keep food washed away from the teeth, and neutralize the decay-causing acids that are produced by plaque bacteria. When the saliva flow is reduced, not only do harmful bacteria grow in the mouth but the gum tissue gets irritated, painful, and more susceptible to periodontal disease. Dry mouth contributes to bad breath and causes dentures to become less stable because they are not able to properly adhere to the tissue in the mouth. More than 400 prescribed and over-the-counter medications cause dry mouth.

Artificial saliva is usually recommended to help alleviate dry mouth. Increasing fluid intake and using sugarless lozenges also help to stimulate saliva. People who have dry mouth must take care of their teeth and gums to minimize the risk of decay and periodontal disease. In addition to regular checkups your dentist may recommend the use of a fluoride mouth rinse or gel to be used in conjunction with preventive care at home.

Dental Decay

Recent studies show that over 60 percent of adults over 65 years of age have tooth root decay. Root caries is more common in the elderly because periodontal disease results in receding gums that leave the softer root surface exposed and susceptible to decay. This problem can be easily prevented by using artificial saliva and fluoride products. It is important to brush with an ADA-approved fluoride toothpaste, use fluoride mouth rinse, floss regularly, and get regular checkups. If you need to have areas of root decay treated, the new bonding techniques can not only match the color of your natural tooth but also protect non-decayed root surfaces that are exposed by receding gum tissue.

Osteoporosis

This disease threatens one out of every twelve Americans. Half of all women and one out of every eight men over 50 years of age suffer a fracture that is attributed to osteoporosis. Studies show 10 to 15 percent of Americans have reduced bone density by age 25. However, significant reductions in density usually don't occur until after age 40. By age 90 about 40 percent of the bone mass is usually lost due to osteoporosis. The disease is more prevelant in white and Asian women than in African Americans. The risk seems greater in women who have early menopause, a family history of the disease, and are small-framed with fair skin. Osteoporosis is called the "silent disease" because it is usually not diagnosed until either a fracture occurs or a loss of skeletal height is noted. Studies show it is influenced by gender, age, genetics, and physical condition. Other factors implicated in the disease are cigarette smoking, excessive alcohol intake, and a high consumption of caffeine, and certain medications for seizures, asthma, arthritis, and elevated thyroid levels. However, the actual mechanisms that cause the disease are not completely understood.

From the dental standpoint, osteoporosis in the elderly leads to resorption of the *alveolar bone*, either causing or following tooth loss. (The alveolar bone supports the teeth in the jaw.) It also contributes to an increase in the risk of fractures during oral surgery and temporo-mandibular disorders in mature and elderly people. In addition, it contributes to the success or failure of implants and the progression of specific forms of periodontal (gum) disease.

Prevention, rather than treatment, is the most successful way to manage osteoporosis. A key to avoiding osteoporosis is to build strong bones, especially before age 35. Regular weight-bearing exercise and resistance training, calcium and vitamin D supplements, and horomone replacement (estrogen) for postmenopausal women are all thought to play a role in the prevention of this disease. According to Dr. Aurelia Nattiv, codirector of the University of California, Los Angeles, Osteoporosis Center, the ideal regimen of calcium for postmenopausal women is 1500 mg a day. For optimal absorption, she suggests calcium citrate tablets be taken between meals, and calcium carbonate tablets should be taken with meals. She also suggests women who don't get out in the sun often, have osteoporosis, or have a family history of the disease take 400 to 800 IU of vitamin D daily.

Treatments for this disease include Alendronate (a biphosphonate) and Calcitonin. Sodium fluoride has been used in patients with spinal fractures because it stimulates bone formation in the vertebrae.

Medication Side Effects

Oral health is closely associated with general health. The natural aging process puts older adults at greater risk for oral health problems because they experience declining physical and/or mental status, exposure to medications for age-related systemic conditions, and reluctance to seek routine dental care.

Studies have shown that people over 65 years of age account for at least one-third of all prescription drug use. Elderly patients seeking dental treatment are presenting medical histories that are increasingly more complex. Medications are a concern for the elderly because they can not only alter the body's defense mechanisms, but also the body's physiologic, immunologic, and biochemical status. When elderly patients present themselves for dental treatment they are likely to be on multiple drug regimens, so the health professional will need to avoid complex drug regimens because they are costly, patient compliance is decreased at this age, and the chance for adverse drug reactions and interactions is greatly increased in this population. It is mandatory for dentists to have a comprehensive medical history before treatment or medications are prescribed. Elderly patients should furnish a list of all medications they are taking and their dosage to dentists before treatment is started. Many dentists will want to contact the patient's primary physician and any other involved professionals before treatment is started, so bring this information with you on your first visit to the dentist's office.

Medications taken by patients are responsible for dry mouth and other salivary gland problems; abnormal bleeding when brushing or flossing; gingival overgrowth; inflammed or ulcerated tissues; microflora imbalance; mouth burning, numbness, or tingling; movement disorders; soft tissue alteration; and taste alteration (see table).

Many of the medications commonly prescribed to elderly patients have both systemic effects and produce adverse reactions in the oral cavity. If an antibiotic is necessary, by all means take it as directed. However, if diarrhea, especially bloody stools, occurs, call your dentist immediately. Elderly patients do not absorb antibiotics as readily as younger patients. Colon problems are not limited to elderly patients, but they are more frequent in that population. Many anti-inflammatory drugs cause gastric irritation, and may produce ulcers.

The drugs most commonly prescribed to the elderly are for treatment of cardiovascular disease. In this group, diurectics used to manage hypertension and drugs from the nitrate group used to treat anginal symptoms can cause dry mouth. Many antihistamines also contribute to dry mouth and eyes. Coumadin, a drug used to treat stroke victims, is

MEDICAL SIDE EFFECTS

ABNORMAL BLEEDING

aspirin	NSAIDs
dipyridamole	warfarin sodium
heparin	

GINGIVAL OVERGROWTH

cyclosporine	nifedipine
diltiazem	phenytoin

INFLAMED OR ULCERATED TISSUES

barbiturates	thiouracil
chloramphenicol	tolbutamide
phenothiazines	trimethadione
quinine	
sulfonamides	

MOUTH BURNING, NUMBNESS, AND TINGLING

antibacterial drugs	oral hypo-
beta blockers	glycemics
hydralazine	tricyclic anti-
	depressants

SOFT TISSUE ALTERATION (discoloration, glossitis, stomatitis, ulceration)

ampicillin	meprobamate
anticoagulants	methyldopa
aspirin	NSAIDs
barbiturates	penicillamine
captopril	phenylbutazone
chloral hydrate	salicylates
cytotoxic agents	sulfonamides
gold compounds	tetracycline
indomethacin	zomepirac
isoniazid	

DRY MOUTH (XEROSTOMIA)

antidepressants	bronchodilators
antihistamines	cough/cold
antihypertensives	preparations
anti-Parkinson drugs	cytotoxic agents
antipsychotics	diuretics
antispasmodics/	phenylbutazone
anticholinergics	scopolamine
atropine	triiodothyronine
barbiturates	

MICROFLORA (BACTERIA) IMBALANCE

antibiotics (long term)	systemic and
cyclosporin	inhaled steroids
insulin	systemic corti-
oral hypo-	costeroids
glycemics	tamoxifen

MOVEMENT DISORDERS

amoxapine	lithium
antipsychotics	metoclopramide
levodopa	

TASTE ALTERATION

Allopurinol	enalapril
azathioprine	ethchlorvynol
baclofen	gold salts
captopril	griseofulvin
carbamazepine	guanethidine
carbencillin	levodopa
chloral hydrate	metronidazole
chlorhexidine	phenylbutazone
diltiazem	sulfaslazine
d-penicillamine	vitamin D

an anticoagulant that can cause bleeding problems when dental treatment is performed. Invasive treatment should not be done without close monitoring of bleeding times. Spontaneous bleeding in the mouth indicates overdosage.

Some antibiotics, such as tetracycline, can be inactivated when taken with antacids. Since many elderly patients take multiple medications and over-the-counter (OTC) items, they need to list on their health history all items (prescribed or OTC) before they see the dentist for treatment.

Aspirin is commonly taken for arthritic conditions. Some doses are near toxic levels. A reaction could be precipitated if the dentist were to prescribe one of the many common aspirin-containing medications to a patient who was already taking large doses of aspirin. If this is a possibility, it should be discussed with your dentist. It is generally recommended that aspirin intake be stopped one week prior to invasive dental treatment.

Codeine-containing analgesics are commonly prescribed for oral pain. Codeine is also constipating. Patients should discuss this problem with their dentist and/or pharmacist before having any prescription filled.

Your dentist should know about heart disease, heart valve damage, joint replacements, and bypass operations before he starts your treatment. Some of these conditions might require antibiotic coverage as suggested by the American Heart Association *before* treatment is started.

In general, the half-life of most drugs is increased in the elderly population. The diminished microsomal enzyme activity in the liver makes the metabolism of drugs slower, and excretion is prolonged because of decreased renal clearance. This results in an increased duration of drug action in the elderly, making the chances of drug interactions and adverse drug reactions higher in this population.

FLUORIDE

The consumer reaction to the issue of fluoridation of the public water supply ranges from gratitude to total outrage. For the purposes of this book, the authors will take the position advocated by the following supporters of fluoridating public water in the United States: the American Dental Association (ADA), the American Cancer Society, the American Heart Association (AHA), American Medical Association (AMA), the Environmental Protection Agency (EPA), the Mayo Clinic, the National Education Association, the U.S. Department of Health and Human Services, the U.S. Public Health Service (PHS), and virtually every other major American health organization. This is a very impressive list of supporters.

The latest census (1992) taken by the Center for Disease Control and Prevention showed 62 percent of Americans using public water supplies enjoyed the benefits of fluoride. (Ninety percent of the population uses public water.) There are now nine states that mandate fluoridation (California, Illinois, South Dakota, Michigan, Ohio, Minnesota, Nebraska, Connecticut, and Georgia). In addition, over 39 countries have chosen to fluoridate their water supplies. Fluoridated table salt has been introduced as a successful alternative method of fluoridation in Ecuador, Switzerland, Colombia, and Mexico, and the rate of caries has dropped 50 percent. Valid scientific studies have clearly shown that fluoride does significantly reduce dental caries with no known side effects to your health.

W. H. Bowen has stated that "caries is clearly an infectious disease." Caufield et al. reported it is spread by kissing and contact with caries-contaminated objects. Studies show fluoride prevents caries by becoming incorporated into the enamel surfaces both before and after a tooth erupts. It also reduces the growth of plaque bacteria that builds up on the teeth and eventually causes caries. Although fluoride is effective in preventing caries on both smooth and irregular surfaces of the teeth, it is most effective on the smooth surfaces of the teeth. Therefore, combining fluoride with pit-and-fissure sealants is a logical combination for optimal protection. After eruption, the most important sources of fluoride are ADA-approved, fluoride-containing toothpastes, mouth rinses, professionally applied topicals, and drinking water. It should be noted that if your water is fluoridated no other fluoride-containing products need be ingested. If your communal water is not fluoridated and has a suboptimal amount of natural fluoride in it, the ADA recommends that your dentist or physician should prescribe fluoride tablets or drops for you and your children to take daily. Before prescribing a fluoride supplement for a child, the health professional needs to know the child's

SUPPLEMENTAL FLUORIDE DOSAGE SCHEDULE
(in milligrams F Per Day*)

Age (years)	Concentration of fluoride in the water (ppm)		
	Less than 0.3	0.3 to 0.6	Greater than 0.6
Birth to 6 months	0	0	0
6 months to 3 years	0.25	0	0
3 years to 6 years	0.5	0.25	0
6 years and up	1.0	0.5	0

* 2.2 mg NaF contains 1 mg F.

age and the concentration of fluoride in the child's "primary" source of drinking water. It should be noted that when fluoride is combined with vitamins the effectiveness of the fluoride is neither enhanced nor reduced.

The ADA recommends fluoride containing dentifrices for people of all ages, whether they live in a fluoridated or nonfluoridated area. It is recommended that very young children be monitored by parents when brushing to insure the toothpaste is not ingested. It is recommended that only a pea-size portion of the dentifrice be put on the brush. Flavored toothpastes that encourage ingestion by young children are discouraged. It is always very important to look for the ADA Seal of Acceptance on products before you purchase them. This means the product has been evaluated by the ADA Council of Scientific Affairs and has demonstrated satisfactory safety and effectiveness. At this writing, three fluoride formulations (NaF, MFP, and SnF2) have received ADA acceptance. It should be noted there are products on the market without the ADA Seal of Acceptance that contain fluoride that is inactive and ineffective.

When fluoride is added to the water system or applied to teeth, studies clearly show it causes remineralization (hardening) of soft areas in the enamel that otherwise would be prone to decay. Studies suggest that continuous exposure to fluoride two to three times a day, on the enamel surfaces of both adult and children's teeth, helps arrest and heal early carious lesions and prevents new ones from developing. The fluoride is stored on the teeth and in plaque. During an acid attack, the fluoride ions are released, making them available at sites that might be demineralizing (becoming prone to caries). It is important to note that early systemic intake of fluoride does not provide lifetime protection.

Many adults are on medications that cause dryness of the mouth (xerostomia), which makes them more prone to tooth decay. Also, older adults often have gum recession. In other words, their gums will recede, causing more tooth surface to be exposed. Fluoride has been shown to help prevent this type of decay. Nearly 40 million adults in the United States are affected by tooth hypersensitivity due to exposed root surfaces. Research indicates that the sensitivity is greatly reduced after topical fluoride is applied. However, the desensitizing effects tend to be short-lived. Now studies show that using fluoride resin in a composite (tooth-colored) restoration gives long-lasting elimination of sensitivity.

Research has shown that after professionally applied gels in a tray are used for four minutes, the fluoride absorbed in the enamel is greater than after exposure for one or two minutes. Therefore, the ADA does not recognize a one-minute application as an acceptable substitute for a four-minute application. Self-applied, ADA-approved fluoride gels are beneficial to patients with a high caries activity, orthodontic appliances, salivary flow problems caused by drugs or radiation therapy, and hypersensitive teeth. The most benefit comes from using these products just before bedtime. The user should restrain from eating or drinking for 30 minutes after the application.

Both prescription and non-prescription over-the-counter, ADA-approved fluoride mouth rinses are now available. Many dental offices use the two-part rinses of APF and SnF2 solutions (used sequentially or in combination) because they are so convenient. However, these rinses have not been tested in large-scale clinical studies. Their concentrations are from 11 to 13 times as much fluoride as the 0.2 percent NaF mouth rinse that has been used by dentists for many years. At this writing, the two-part rinses have not been recognized or approved by the American Dental Association or the Food and Drug Administration.

It is recommended that for home use the over-the-counter fluoride rinses be used after brushing at bedtime. They should be swished vigorously once a day for one minute and expectorated. For maximum benefit, patients should not rinse, eat, or drink for 30 minutes after they are used.

Fluoride varnishes have been used in Europe and Canada for 20 years to prevent caries. A fluoride varnish, Duraflor, recently received Food and Drug Administration approval for use in the United States. Fluoride varnishes offer the advantage of prolonged contact of fluoride to the teeth. They form a film on the teeth that hardens on contact with saliva. After four hours, the varnish is removed by brushing thoroughly. Clinical studies indicate professionally applied solutions and gels are still superior in caries prevention.

January 1995 marked the 50th anniversary of communal water fluoridation, and about 165 million people use fluoridated water sources today. Studies show that children who drink water containing the proper amount of fluoride (1.0 to 1.5 milligrams per liter [mg/1]; optimally, 1.2 mg/1) from birth can expect 60 percent fewer cavities. Many supplies of drinking water contain well in excess of the optimal amount of 1.2 mg/1 of fluoride. Studies have shown that dental *fluorosis* can occur in water with fluoride levels of more than 2 mg/1. Fluorosis is a discoloration of the teeth that is usually unnoticable to most people. It is characterized by lacy white lines or mottling (discolored blotches), and pitting of teeth. The position of the U.S. Surgeon General is that "fluorosis is a cosmetic rather than a health problem." The ADA has supported this position.

The EPA states that the element fluorine (a gas) is so universal that it ranks 17th in abundance of the earth's elements, 13th in the human body, and 12th in the earth's oceans. In fact, sea water contains 1.4 mg/1 fluoride. It is very interesting to note that 1.4 mg/1 in sea water is very near the ideal concentration recommended for drinking water, 1.2 mg/1.

The ADA states that fluoridation of drinking water returns a 20-fold return in dollars saved in repairing decayed teeth. The per capita expense of fluoridation in a large community over a lifetime comes to about 12 cents a year. In addition, studies indicate that of the substances used to make water safe and suitable for human consumption, "none has been more thoroughly researched than fluoride, nor proven to have a better safety record." Drinking adequately fluoridated water represents one of the most economical preventive values in the nation.

The National Institute of Dental Research in Bethesda, Maryland, has been working on a very unique method of fluoride delivery. It involves a tiny disk about the width of an aspirin and half its thickness that can be bonded with an acid-etch material to a back molar. An active "time release" fluoride compound, which would be released continuously at a rate of one milligram of fluoride per day, is contained in this disk. Recent studies indicate this amount is considered ideal.

The continuous release of fluoride could reduce dental caries, reverse the early stages of dental caries, and prevent future dental caries. The beauty of the system is that it would allow each person to make their own decision about participating, and it would be monitored by a dental professional, probably a dentist. The fluoride disks could be replaced when necessary to insure their continuing action.

It would seem that there is enough fluoride around to eliminate the need for dentists to repair teeth. This thought could fast become a reality.

SEDATION AND PSYCHOSEDATION: ORAL, NITROUS OXIDE/OXYGEN, AND INTRAVENOUS

The use of oral sedation, nitrous oxide/oxygen, and intravenous (IV) sedation as an adjunct to dental treatment are helpful in allaying the fear and blocking the memory of dental treatment, as well as allowing the patient relaxation. None is without risk. Dentists are generally of the opinion that, when properly administered, the use of oral sedation or nitrous oxide/oxygen is very safe. The use of intravenous drugs should only be used by those dentists who have training in addition to that received during the four years of dental school. When considering sedation, the patient must be fully informed of the risks of the drugs to be used and have the opportunity to weigh the risks against the potential benefits of their use.

Oral sedation offers a way to reduce dental anxiety without all the risks of being "put out." Valium, Librium, Paxipam, Xanax, and Halcion are each used for this purpose. These drugs have basically the same effect as conscious sedation without nearly the risk involved with putting the drug directly into the bloodstream. Advocates of intravenous sedation argue that oral sedation is not as predictable as IV sedation because of the differing tolerance levels of patients to the various drugs. However, after over 25 years of patient care, I have yet to find a patient, other than an habitual drug user, whose apprehension I could not "Take the edge off" by using oral sedation.

I do not want to imply that oral sedation is without potential risks. However, the absorption of drugs orally is slower and, hence, safer as a general rule. Any drug reaction would usually come about more slowly, thus making it more manageable. Drugs induced directly into the bloodstream travel much faster through the body. Oral sedation accomplishes the same end result as "conscious sedation," the relief of extreme patient anxiety.

Oral sedation is usually given to the patient thirty minutes to one hour before their dental appointment. It usually takes about three hours for the effect to diminish. The dosage is based on the weight and age of the patient. Very anxious patients are sometimes given enough of the medication to take at bedtime the night before their dental appointment to insure they get a good night's rest. Early morning appointments are usually best for these patients to keep their anxiety level as low as possible.

Nitrous oxide (laughing gas) is a colorless, odorless gas which when inhaled can cause euphoria, amnesia, and/or slight analgesia. It is mixed with oxygen to prevent asphyxiation or overdose. An inhalation mask is placed over the nose of the patient. As the patient breathes in through the nose only, the effects of drowsiness, floating, and euphoria are felt. The extent of the effects can be controlled by varying the percentage of nitrous oxide in the inhaled gas. Nitrous concentrations of 50 to 60 percent are routinely used in the dental office. It is a consensus of opinion that either the doctor or a staff member with training in nitrous oxide/oxygen sedation should be with the patient at all times when they are on nitrous oxide/oxygen sedation. *Patients should never be left alone.* It is usually suggested that the patient be given 100 percent oxygen for five to ten minutes before dismissing to flush the nitrous oxide out of his system. This will keep the patient from getting a headache. There are some reports of patients experiencing nausea and sexual hallucinations as a result of this sedation.

This method of anxiety control has the advantage of being totally reversible at the end of the appointment so that the patient is in a normal state before leaving the dental office.

Intravenous sedation for dental treatment is a serious procedure that involves potentially life-threatening risks. For this reason, I feel the administration of IV sedation at any dental appointment should be the exception, rather than the rule. Exceptions might be a person who is a dental phobic (a person with an irrational fear), a handicapped person who otherwise could not receive treatment, or a patient who needs extensive dental treatment or surgery.

Dentists have the option of suggesting to patients with anxiety that they can either have oral sedation, nitrous oxide/oxygen, or seek psychological treatment (in extreme cases) for their dental phobia rather than using IV sedation. Studies using relaxation and desensitizing techniques also have had very successful results.

Discuss your alternatives with your dentist. You may find that knowing, trusting, and talking to him goes a long way toward relieving anxiety.

When using IV sedation, one or more of the following drugs may be used: Versed, Decadron, Inapsine, Atropine, Nembutal, Demerol, Scopolamine, or Valium. The risks involved when using these drugs are that they may cause respiratory and/or cardiac failure or an allergic reaction. Any or all of these complications could be fatal. Proper dosage of these drugs is determined by the person administering the drug through observing the signs and symptoms exhibited by the patient. Almost without exception, most authorities agree that there should *always* be one person responsible for the administration of the anesthesia and monitoring the patient, and another person responsible for performing the dental treatment. I would *never* advise you to allow a dentist to treat you if he does not have another person who is properly trained to administer the IV sedation and monitor your vital signs (blood pressure, breathing, pulse and heart rates, temperature, etc.). In many cases, when death or brain damage occur as a result of IV sedation, the cause has been inadequate patient monitoring. Unless the dentist does IV sedations on a regular basis, he will usually need to see you at a hospital or in a surgery clinic in order to have the properly trained personnel, life support equipment, etc. available in case of an emergency. Patients are usually fully recovered within a few hours after the procedure is completed, and are able to go home.

If you are unsure about using IV sedation for a dental procedure you need to check with several dentists in your area to see if they would use IV sedation for the same procedure. Because of the concern for patient's safety, many states today require a dentist to have special training before he administers IV sedation. Almost all insurance companies have guidelines for covering dentists who administer IV sedation, and the premiums charged for coverage of this procedure are much higher.

In August 1985, the ADA developed a policy regarding IV sedation for state dental organizations. In general, the policy called for "formal continuing education for the use of conscious sedation techniques and a one-year minimum advanced education program for the use of 'deep sedation' and general anesthesia." The ADA statement also called for each individual state to establish their own educational requirements and to conduct on-site office inspections for offices of dentists using IV sedation on patients.

Most regulations that have been instituted distinguish between general anesthesia (or unconscious sedation) and conscious sedation. *General anesthesia* (or *unconscious sedation*) describes a state whereby the patient is not responsive to verbal commands, and his vital signs (e.g. breathing) may need support. *Conscious sedation* implies that the patient is responsive to voice commands and should not require any life support to maintain him. There is a very fine line between these two types of sedation. An additional small increment of an injected drug used for conscious sedation can produce general anesthesia. Herein lies the danger!

The reason surrounding this controversy is that many states had no guidelines for the use of IV sedation in dental offices. As a result, some dentists were taking continuing education courses that lasted several weeks and others were taking courses that only lasted a short time (a few days). Many states also did not have any guidelines for equipment and medications necessary for life support systems in the office setting. Most authorities agreed more stringent guidelines were needed.

In California, the prototype for much dental legislation, representatives from all five dental schools in that state agreed that "no less than 150 hours" of anesthesia training should be necessary for a dentist to administer IV sedation in the state of California. That is less than four weeks of training if one assumes eight hours of training per day. However, other faculty members in California dental schools and dentists in private practice feel strongly that even more hours of training are necessary. The controversy still exists. You can call your state dental society (see the appendix in the back of this book) to find out the guidelines in your state. I feel this is an instance where consumer groups could and should become involved with state dental boards.

Regardless of whether IV or oral sedation is used, your dentist should be sure that when you leave his office you have a responsible adult to accompany you home, that you have written postoperative instructions, and that you have a telephone number to call in case of any type of emergency that might arise postoperatively. These details should be worked out prior to treatment.

DENTISTRY FOR THE HANDICAPPED PATIENT

The term "handicapped" encompasses a wide range of mental, physical, and/or medical impairments. The degree of impairment, in many instances, depends to a great extent on the patient's attitude. The extremely handicapped are confined to beds in hospitals, nursing homes, or private homes. Others are confined to wheelchairs because they are amputees, paralyzed, or too heavily medicated to stand, walk, or function on their own without potentially injuring themselves. Some are emotionally fragile and must be treated with extreme love, care, understanding, and patience. Many of these patients are undergoing psychiatric care and are heavily tranquilized. Many patients, both young and old, are on multiple medications for chronic debilitating diseases of the heart, liver, or other organs.

All of these patients deserve and need the same quality of dental care as the nonhandicapped patients, including restoring or crowning carious (decayed) teeth; treating periodontal disease; checking for oral cancer; and, perhaps most importantly, teaching dental disease preventive techniques. Home care is one of the most important aspects of the handicapped patient's dental needs. Patients who have dexterity problems or a physical disability may have difficulty holding onto their toothbrush or dental floss. It may be helpful to try some of the following:

1. Attach the toothbrush to your hand with a wide elastic rubberband.
2. Use a rubber ball, bicycle handle grip, or a sponge to enlarge the handle of the toothbrush. Also try winding adhesive tape or an elastic bandage around the handle of the brush.
3. The handle of the toothbrush can be lengthened by securing with tape a piece of wood or plastic such as a ruler, tongue depressor, or popsicle stick. The handle can be bent by running hot water over the handle (not the head) of the toothbrush.
4. It is easier to handle floss if it is tied into a loop before using.
5. Electric toothbrushes and commercial floss holders are easier to use.

For some handicapped patients squeezing toothpaste from a tube onto a toothbrush is a major task because they do not have full use of their hands and/or arms. It is also difficult for some to brush adequately. Even though handicapped patients want to be self-sufficient, many often have to depend on nurses or other helping "partners" to perform their everyday tasks. Unfortunately, the responsible "partners" do not always know the dental needs of their charges. Whenever possible, a dentist should speak to these partners and explain the basics of home care. For example, many handicapped patients use a 9 percent fluoride solution as a substitute for toothpastes. For patients with dry mouth, glycerine is swabbed on the gingiva to keep it from becoming dry and irritated. Custom-made devices are often attached to the wheelchair lock handle so handicapped patients can use them to brush, write, etc.

Many handicapped patients must be seen in their own environment, rather than in the conventional dental office setting. To insure better care for patients in nursing homes, Congress passed the Medicare and Medicaid Nursing Home Reform Provisions of the Omnibus Budget Reconciliation Act of 1987. This legislation mandates that routine and emergency dental services be available to all nursing home residents. In order to obtain Medicare and Medicaid certification, these facilities must comply with the act, and they are monitored by regular inspections that include interviews with the residents. In addition to the federal standards, nursing homes are also subject to state licensure requirements, which are usually more stringent and comprehensive.

Dental care in nursing home facilities requires the involvement of not only the dentist and his staff, but also the facility's staff. The staff needs to be trained in proper cleaning techniques for both natural dentition and dentures. Before considering a nursing home, it is a good idea to ask residents about their experiences with dental care while there. If they have had a new denture made or an existing one repaired, find out how long it took and if they were satisfied. Ask what provisions are in place for seeing a dentist on an emergency basis. Find out if the staff is actively involved in the daily routine care needs of the oral health of the residents.

Some dentists have literally "hit the road" with mobile offices. They go to the homes of those who cannot come to them. The availability of a wide array of mobile dental equipment has made mobile dentistry very popular and accessible. Many times this mode of dental delivery is under the auspices of community-based programs, dental schools, or other nonprofit ventures. Your local dental society can tell you if such a service is available in your community.

In 1990 the Americans with Disabilities Act (AwDA) was passed. It mandates that health care providers make "public accommodations" available to the disabled and provide equal access to services. Barrier-free access to the dentist's office, the treatment rooms, and the restroom facilities are required in order to be in compliance with the law.

Other important considerations for handicapped patients include scheduling convenient appointments, providing written post-treatment instructions, and a dental staff prepared to handle particular needs (including any possible emergency situation).

For information, or help in locating a dentist, the following groups may be helpful.

Academy of Dentistry for the Handicapped
211 East Chicago Avenue
Chicago, Illinois 60611
(312) 440-2660

National Foundation of Dentistry for the Handicapped
1600 Stout Street, Suite 1420
Denver, Colorado 80202
(303) 573-0264

American Dental Association
211 East Chicago Avenue
Chicago, Illinois 60611
(312) 440-2500

American Academy of Pediatric Dentistry
211 East Chicago Avenue, Suite #1036
Chicago, Illinois 60611
(312) 337-2169

The Grottoes of North America
Dentistry for the Handicapped
34 N. Fourth Street
Columbus, Ohio 43215
(614) 463-9193

National Oral Health Information Clearinghouse
1 NOHIC Way
Bethesda, Maryland 20892-3500
(301) 402-7364
(301) 907-8830 (fax)

DENTAL FEAR

Most people don't like going to the dentist. Some even approach their dentist by stating, "I hate dentists." Actually, they don't hate dentists; they are fearful of the treatment their dentist renders to them. A person who is a true dental phobic may carry their fear to extremes by taking extra-long routes to and from work, just to avoid driving by the dentist's office. A landmark study published in 1984 by Drs. Scott, Hirshman, and Schroder reported that up to 80 percent of the population experience some degree of dental fear, and extreme dental fear is a problem for every one in four patients. For 10 to 12 million true dental phobics in the United States, fears may be so extreme that they will seek dental treatment only when they have severe pain and major problems.

Anxious dental patients many times repeatedly cancel their appointments, arrive late knowing they will have to be rescheduled, or just don't show at all. This results in a progressive deterioration of their dental health. When treatment is rendered, these patients many times are not in control of their emotions, are not cooperative, and certainly are not stoical about pain. *These patients usually don't stop to realize that their behavior makes the dentist, his staff, and any other patients in the office very anxious.* The result may be substandard treatment.

Research indicates that fear of the unknown, loss of control, bodily injury, and helplessness and dependency are the four elements common to fears and phobias. Anxious patients report that dental injections and drilling are the two most feared procedures that occur in the dental office. Try to identify your specific fears and concerns. Many times patients' fears have been traced to parents who preconditioned them as children to be afraid. Preconditioning usually happens subtly, though sometimes it may be all too obvious. For example, a mother might say, "Johnny, if you are not good, I am going to take you to the dentist so he can take out all of your teeth."

Stories (real or not) that we all hear about the horrors that have occurred at the hands of some dentist also have a great influence. Many times, the person relating the story has actually gone through a frightening experience that has left a lifelong mark. It is important to understand that our dental fears are not unique and, most important, that there are ways to control these feelings.

If you experience dental anxiety, it is important for you to recognize your anxiety, accept it as a common reaction to an uncertain situation, and learn to master it. This will help you be more comfortable about dental visits, which in turn will boost your confidence and oral health.

Dental fear is usually managed by either pharmacological or behavioral methods. Hypnotic or anti-anxiety drugs can either be administered orally, intravenously, or a mixture of nitrous oxide/oxygen may be inhaled. Pain is controlled primarily by topical anesthetic gels (or solutions) and injectable anesthetic solutions. Hypnotic or anti-anxiety drugs administered orally or intravenously may also block pain responses.

Patients can be tranquilized with medications such as Valium, and the pain is controlled with topical and local anesthesia, conscious sedation (nitrous oxide/oxygen, "laughing gas"), and general anesthesia (IV sedation). Even though these methods are beneficial, they carry a risk. Anytime pharmacological methods are used to control pain there is always the risk of side effects, not to mention the danger of fostering dependence on the medications.

Pain relief through the use of behavioral management eliminates the risk of dependence. Some of these methods include biofeedback, hypnosis, and progressive relaxation techniques. Anxiety relief through the use of behavioral management eliminates the risk of drug dependence.

The logical approach to eliminate fear is to treat the cause, not just the symptoms, but efforts in this regard are just beginning in dentistry. Psychotherapists use desensitization techniques to help patients with all types of fears and anxieties, and that includes dental fears, too. The most successful method involves the patient developing a list of all the most frightening aspects of treatment. He or she then organizes the list starting with the least frightening and progressing to the most frightening. Patients are asked to try to associate each situation in their minds with a pleasant experience and to think for several minutes about each pairing. When one situation no longer brings on feelings of anxiety, the patient moves on to the next item until all have been dealt with. This process is best done under the supervision of a trained therapist.

Another method involves distracting oneself from the procedures by, for example, listening to a relaxing tape or going over shopping lists. In yet another technique, apprehensive patients are trained to concentrate on breathing at the rate of eight breaths per minute. This relaxation exercise keeps the patient's attention focused on something other than the dental treatment. Another common relaxation technique involves systematically tightening and then relaxing the major muscle groups in your legs, arms, hands, neck, and shoulders.

Using visualization is an excellent way to feel more relaxed and comfortable before and after a dental visit. For instance, before your visit you can visualize yourself sitting calmly in the dentist's chair while he is examining your mouth or restoring your tooth. You can also focus on a relaxing scene from your favorite vacation spot or activity and hold it before your "mind's eye" during treatment.

One of the best ways of handling dental fears is also the simplest: Communication between the dentist and you. Before you go for treatment share your feelings with the dentist and his staff. Let them know you are fearful, tense, or anxious so they can tailor their treatment and their pace to your needs. If you know what is going on and can make your needs known, it will help you feel less helpless and anxious. The dentist should fully explain each step of the dental examination or procedure to you. The more you know about the reasons for a certain procedure and what will be done during it, the more confident and relaxed you will feel. You, in turn, should ask those questions that will help allay your fears. Knowledge helps you to gain control over an unfamiliar situation and enables you to choose comfortably between the treatment options recommended by your dentist. This is a good beginning and has the highest probability of resulting in a positive experience for both you and your dentist. Ways to improve communication include developing hand signals to indicate a need for a break, the fact that anesthesia is not adequate, or your wish to stop treatment for that day.

If these signals are agreed upon before treatment starts, you will feel more secure and in control.

Always schedule your dental visit at a stress-free time when you won't be rushed, physically strained, or troubled by other concerns. You may find a Saturday or early morning appointment less stressful than trying to rush to see the dentist directly from work. Always get a good night's sleep and eat a light meal before your appointment. Dress in comfortable, loose clothes. If possible, schedule short dental appointments by having different procedures performed on different days.

Keep in mind that when you see a dentist on a regular basis most of your visits will involve preventive measures—examining and cleaning your teeth and X rays. This will give you an opportunity to get acquainted with the dentist and his staff, which will help you feel comfortable and relaxed. Sometimes it helps to take a friend or family member who has a positive attitude toward dental care with you.

The dentist-patient relationship is a mutual one between you and your dentist. Get into the habit of thinking of yourself as an active participant in your dental care. You will be glad you did, and you'll come away smiling.

LASERS IN DENTISTRY

A laser is a tube or sealed cavity into which either a gas or crystal is placed. One end of the tube has a mirror that is fully reflective, and the other end has a partially transmissive mirror. When the laser is turned on a source of energy is created inside the tube. This creates a spontaneous and stimulated emission called the *laser beam*. The beam of light does not diverge and has one wavelength. Lasers are set apart from other light-generation sources because of their ability to emit concentrated energy that is collimated (focused with no scattering), allowing for the use of precision optics to transmit the generated energy.

There is no single laser that can do all procedures, since each type of laser works at different wavelengths and each of these wavelengths reacts differently with different tissues. Therefore, it is important to use the most appropriate type of laser for the procedure. Laser technology has been quickly accepted in ophthalmology and other surgical disciplines because it enables procedures to be performed that have not been possible using conventional methods. However, most procedures in dentistry that can be performed with lasers can also be performed by using other more conventional methods. Prior to 1990, the only laser available on the dental market was the first-generation CO_2 laser with straight beams that were transmitted through hollow articulated arms with mirrors in them. It was nearly impossible to use this laser in the back of the mouth. Currently there are four types of lasers that have received FDA clearance in the United States for soft-tissue use. They are the CO_2 laser (now in its second generation), the Nd:YAG laser, the argon laser–green wavelength, and the Ho:YAG laser.

Lasers have been clinically proven and FDA-approved in the United States for a wide range of soft-tissue uses. Some of the uses include:

1. tissue reduction and contouring (e.g. gingivectomies [surgical removal of pockets], crown lenghtening, frenectomies [surgical removal of attachment tissue under the tongue or the midline of the lip], and second-stage exposure of implants)
2. coagulation of bleeding areas
3. biopsies
4. symptomatic relief of mouth ulcers
5. oral infection therapy

Another use the FDA in the United States has approved for lasers is to use them to cure composite restorative material (argon laser–blue wavelength).

And just recently the FDA approved lasers for use on hard tissue (bone and teeth). This does not, however, include removal of a amalgam. Worldwide, dental lasers have been used to vaporize caries (decay), eliminate hypersensitivity, etch enamel, and do root canal therapy by vaporizing pulp (nerve) tissue and condensing gutta percha.

When lasers are used authorities report some universal clinical advantages. For example, lasers greatly reduce bleeding, causing the field to be dry and visibility to be enhanced. Lasers also seal blood vessels and lymphatics, resulting in minimal postoperative swelling. Patients report they experience little to no postoperative pain when lasers are used. Authorities say the reason is the nerve fibers are sealed with the laser light. Lasers also significantly reduce scarring, eliminate the need for sutures (stitches), and cause the bacteria count at the treatment site to be so low that many times the field is actually sterile.

Dental lasers are safe to use if proper precautions are followed. Proper training and knowledge by the dentist and his staff are very important. Each procedure requires the appropriate type of laser be used at the appropriate setting and dosage to reduce the risk of tissue damage. Everyone in the operatory, including the patient, should wear the appropriate protective goggles. Different types of lasers require different types of safety glasses, which should never be interchanged.

Researchers are hoping to develop the technology to use lasers to reduce hypersensitivity in teeth by sealing the *dentinal tubules*, and to eliminate caries (decay) formation in teeth. At this time, there is a relatively small amount of formal, long-term clinical research and documentation. The goal for lasers in the future is to have all the wavelengths incorporated into a single unit to allow a variety of procedures to be accomplished. It is the energy of each wavelength absorbed by the target tissue that brings about the desired effect.

Three main benefits of lasers are that they have an anti-inflammatory effect, promote healing, and reduce pain. The laser can be an important tool when used in conjunction with conventional procedures or as a sole form of treatment, since many problems that cause patients to seek dental treatment involve inflammation and pain.

TOBACCO CESSATION IN DENTISTRY

There are currently 46.3 million citizens in the United States who smoke, and another 12 million who use smokeless tobacco (ST). Statistics show about one quarter of all dental patients use tobacco. It is scientifically recognized that smoking is the nation's leading preventable health problem and is responsible for one in every six deaths in the United States. It is common knowledge there is a link between smoking, lung cancer, and heart disease. Smoking also contributes to cancer of the kidney, cervix, pancreas, bladder, and stomach. From the standpoint of oral health, smoking (cigarette, pipe, and cigar) is linked to cancer of the mouth, pharynx, esophagus, and larynx. Chronic use of smokeless tobacco has been directly linked to cancer of the larynx, mouth, throat, and esophagus. Chronic ST users are 50 times more likely to develop oral cancer than nonusers, and the risks are greatest in intraoral locations where the tobacco is usually stored. Oral cancer is usually treated with a combination of radiation therapy, chemotherapy, and surgery. If it is not diagnosed early, oral cancer may require extensive, disfiguring surgery; or, worse, it may be fatal. The overall five-year survival rate for oral cancer patients is about 50 percent, with only 23 percent of those with regional lymph node involvement surviving.

Leukoplakia is a soft-tissue lesion that is characterized by a white patch or plaque. It is usually a localized condition that is related to irritation from a badly fitting denture, broken teeth, or tobacco. High-risk sites include the floor of the mouth and the underside of the tongue. Although leukoplakia is not exclusively seen in tobacco users, it is definitely associated with both smoking and smokeless tobacco use. The tobacco/leukoplakia association is related to the frequency, amount, and duration of the tobacco use. It has been reported that 2 to 6 percent of leukoplakia will become malignant. Further, the lesions often heal when tobacco use is stopped.

Overwhelming scientific evidence shows *peridontal (gum) disease* is more likely to occur in smokers than nonsmokers, and it is usually more severe (often resulting in tooth loss). It is interesting to note that smokers usually have higher levels of dental plague, but the tendency for their gums to bleed is lower. The diagnosis and treatment of periodontal disease for this group may be delayed because they don't usually have bleeding gums.

The oral effects of smoking are stains on teeth, tooth restorations, and the tongue; calculus buildup on the teeth; and bad breath. Smoking dulls a person's ability to taste and smell; irritates tissues in the mouth; and delays healing after a tooth has been extracted (including a dry socket) or after oral surgery. Several studies have shown that smoking is the greatest barrier to tissue healing after periodontal therapy, especially when soft tissue is grafted and/or surgery is performed. Periodontal therapy is more likely to fail if the patient continues to smoke. There is a positive association between smokeless tobacco use and gingival (gum) tissue recession at the site where the tobacco is usually stored in the mouth. Smoking cessation is usually associated with a reduction in the formation of calculus.

The American Dental Association has launched an all-out effort that will last until the year 2000 to involve dentists in an organized intervention program to provide tobacco-cessation services to patients. It is especially important for periodontists and oral surgeons to be active in this program because periodontal disease, oral cancer, and wound healing are so closely linked to cigarette smoking. Well-trained oral health professionals are able to offer tobacco cessation counseling with minimal interruptions in patients' daily routines. They are the most logical health professional to provide this information to patients because they already see patients on a regular basis each year.

Whatever the reason people give for continuing to smoke, the reality is that nicotine, a drug found in tobacco, is addictive. It is a stimulant that increases the heart rate and blood pressure, and it acts on the pleasure centers deep within the brain. It causes both physical and emotional addiction. As smokers develop a tolerance to nicotine they need more to get the same physiological/psychological effect. This makes their addiction very difficult to overcome.

The FDA has approved prescriptive agents (such as nicotine-containing gum and transdermal patches) to be used in conjunction with tobacco-cessation programs. The ADA has also recently created a new code for oral health professionals to use to bill insurance companies for their counseling services.

If you don't smoke, don't start! If you want to stop, here are some techniques listed in a recent brochure from the ADA:

- Make a list of reasons you want to quit
- Set a date you will quit, and then do it
- Join a formal smoking-cessation support group
- Exercise
- Keep your mouth occupied with sugarless gum, etc.
- Keep your hands occupied with needlepoint, woodworking, etc.
- Choose a low-stress time such as your vacation to stop smoking
- Stop carrying matches and cigarettes
- Stop all at once—cold turkey
- Don't let setbacks discourage you—keep trying!
- Use all available resources (audio and video tapes, books, and self-help materials)
- Ask your dentist or physician for a prescription for FDA-approved products for tobacco cessation

If you need more advice or help call the National Cancer Institute's toll free Cancer Information Service at 1-800-4-CANCER.

LATEX ALLERGY

In the early 1980s dental professionals began wearing gloves on a regular basis to reduce the risk of disease transmission. No one realized at that time how easily the population would become sensitized to latex. Recent statistics indicate about 13.7 percent of dental professionals have latex allergies. The incidence among physicians is 5.6 percent and 7.4 percent for nurses. Dental professionals are especially vulnerable because they are exposed to the material more than other health care workers.

Studies show that there are three main groups of people who are most susceptible to latex allergies. They include individuals with spinal cord deformities (including spina bifida), health professionals, and atopic individuals who have undergone many surgical procedures. Atopy, the tendency to develop some type of allergy, is inherited, but the specific form of allergy is not. Atopy includes hay fever, eczema, asthma, and food allergies (especially bananas or chestnuts). Repeated exposure to an antigen will increase sensitivity to that agent due to the manner in which allergies develop. This explains the high incidence of latex allergy among surgical personnel and individuals who require repeated surgery. Exposure duration also plays a role in latex allergy development. Dental health professionals wear gloves for extended periods of time, so they are the most susceptible to latex allergies. The FDA reports mucous membranes (such as those located inside the mouth) may be especially reactive in the latex sensitive patient. That is why dental professionals are especially concerned about exposing a previously sensitized patient to latex when performing dental procedures.

Researchers have identified that two types of allergens (or antigens) in the latex cause the reactions. They are the proteins (a natural component of latex) and the chemicals used in the manufacturing process to give the gloves strength and elasticity.

There are two possible allergic reactions to natural rubber latex. First, the immediate (Type I) reaction can occur within minutes of exposure. Its symptoms include asthma, edema, eczema, nausea, and anaphylaxis. A severe anaphylactic reaction can cause death within minutes if appropriate action is not taken. The reactions can involve the respiratory and the gastrointestinal tract, and the cardiovascular system.

The delayed (Type IV) hypersensitivity reaction is more common. The initial symptoms are itching, redness, and visicles affecting only the exposed area. After a period of time the skin often dries out and sores can develop. This is called an acquired immune reaction, and it is caused by the chemicals used to make the gloves. Usually it appears about five hours after exposure and peaks 24 to 48 hours after exposure. The most common approach to dealing with this allergy is to ignore it, or use steroid creams to alleviate the symptoms. Unfortunately, this allows the body to build even greater levels of antibodies to latex proteins, allowing the allergy to get worse. Allergies can be difficult to diagnose because the reactions themselves can vary from slight itchiness to cardiovascular collapse leading to shock, depending on the individual.

In 1991, the Food and Drug Administration issued an alert to health professionals to screen patients for latex sensitivity and report any cases found. Patients should be asked questions about adverse reactions to balloons, adhesive tapes, or rubber work gloves or boots. Patients who must wash all rubber products before wearing them should be considered allergic until proven otherwise. Anyone who has an occupational exposure to latex should be questioned carefully. Any patients identified with allergic reactions should be told about latex sensitivity and advised to seek allergy testing. At this writing, the FDA has cleared for marketing a test system to aid in the clinical diagnosis of patients suspected of having a latex allergy; it is not for general screening. The test (Alastat Latex-Specific IgE Allergen Test Kit, Diagnosis Products Corporation, Los Angeles, California) measures circulating levels of immunoglobulin E (IgE) specific to latex (Type I allergy). Until now the diagnosis of Type I latex allergy has been dependent solely on the clinical history and physical examination of the patient. No test or combination of tests is capable of diagnosing with absolute certainty, but this new test will be helpful when combined with other information. The test accurately detected latex sensitivity more than 85 percent of the time in patients with confirmed latex allergy. If the allergy is confirmed, the patient should be told the importance of alerting all health care workers with whom they come into contact about the allergy. Medical identification bracelets are available so emergency medical personnel will be aware of the allergy. Professionals should use items made of alternative materials such as vinyl or plastic on patients with latex allergies. *Hypoallergenic products should not be substituted for latex because they can and do still sometimes initiate an allergic reaction in people allergic to latex.* Currently, devices and materials containing latex are not required to be labeled. Dentists should adopt a protocol to follow for latex-sensitive patients to insure that only non-latex substitutions are used. The FDA is working towards mandating changes in labeling and advertising because materials labeled hypoallergenic have not always prevented adverse latex reactions.

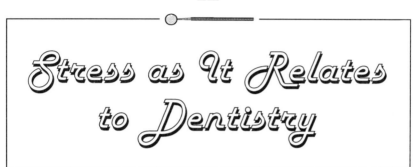

12

Stress as It Relates to Dentistry

In today's fast-paced world it is not uncommon for people to feel a tremendous amount of stress in their daily lives. Many of us cope with stress by exercising or using biofeedback. However, some of us take out our stress on our bodies. Most authorities consider *bruxism* (tooth grinding) and *temporomandibular joint* (TMJ) problems (those related to the hinge joint connecting the lower jaw to the upper jawbone) as directly related to stress.

The only positive cure for bruxism or TMJ problems is to change your lifestyle. Since most of us are not in a position to do this, we have to look to other methods that will help the symptoms. Many general dentists and specialists have become very interested in this area of dentistry. Since little formal training in this area is given in dental schools today, the information is being disseminated to the dental community through continuing education courses.

If you have a problem with bruxism or TMJ you should call the office of an oral and maxillofacial surgeon, a periodontist, a prosthodontist, or your general dentist and explain your situation. One of these dentists should be able to refer you to someone in your area familiar with treating your type of problem. Since there is no simple solution to this type of problem, your treatment could extend over a long period of time. Many people never are able to "cure" their problem, but usually they experience some degree of relief from the symptoms. Now let us look at each of these two problems more closely.

BRUXISM (TOOTH GRINDING)

Bruxism can directly or indirectly cause many problems. Teeth can become painful or loose, and sometimes parts of the teeth are literally ground away. Many times this leaves them with worn surfaces or fractured enamel, making it necessary to restore them with crowns.

Bruxism (grinding your teeth together) eventually causes destruction to the supportive bone and gingiva of the teeth. This can lead to temporomandibular disorder (TMD), to be discussed in the next section. Many people do not realize they even have a problem until their mate comments that they make a horrible grinding sound when they are sleeping.

At this writing there has not been enough research done to determine the exact cause of bruxism, but it is thought that both emotional and physical factors are involved. Some contributing factors are thought to be stress, an abnormal bite, sleep disorders, and crooked or missing teeth.

"People under stress are very likely to grind their teeth," writes Dr. Norma Scott Kinzer in her book, *Stress and the American Woman*. Kinzer, an expert on stress, was codirector of Project Athena, a study of the first female cadets at West Point. Now that is stress!

Kinzer herself admits to being a "champion tooth grinder." She says she is "living testimony to the relationship between stress and high dental bills." In addition, she feels that "tooth grinding is one of the most serious dental problems in the United States today. It is estimated that from 30 to 100 percent of the adult population in the United States grind their teeth. Studies show the problem is most prevalent in young (18–26-year-old) college-age females. Children also brux. They can start as early as three years of age. They usually stop by the age of 12. Adult bruxers usually start about 20 years of age and stop by 40. We still do not know if child bruxers grow up to become adult bruxers. However, bruxism does seem to occur in the same family, so it could be a genetic factor or a response learned from parents as a coping mechanism.

There are a number of ways to treat bruxism. Your dentist will be able to determine which treatment or combination of treatments is best for you. Since stress is thought to be the major cause of bruxism, people need to learn ways to relax. People who are stressed may need to seek counseling. Your dentist can prescribe muscle relaxants to relax jaw muscles. It may be necessary to have physical therapy.

If you grind your teeth it may be helpful to do the following:

1. Break the habit by placing reminders around the house of repeat phrases to help you relax.

2. Apply a warm cloth to the side of your face to help relax the clenched muscles.
3. Stress will be relieved if you cut down on caffeine, take warm baths, and stop being so demanding of yourself.

Many authorities feel that patients who brux may run the risk of other problems, such as those associated with the jaw joint (temporomandibular joint, or TMJ for short) after a prolonged history of the habit. Patients are considered "vicious bruxers" if they develop TMJ problems, headaches, facial pain, fatigue, sore jaw muscles, or severely wear down their teeth. If you develop these symptoms, treatment may be needed.

A *splint* (bite plate) is usually recommended, whether the bruxer is a child or an adult. But splints are usually reserved for cases in which the habit has become destructive to the teeth, muscles, or the TMJ. A splint is a plastic device (usually soft ones are made for children) that fits over the teeth and distributes the forces of grinding equally. Authorities agree that a splint is a good way to manage a bruxer, but it is not a cure.

Modern society places many demands on our lives. Sometimes, we exceed our ability to comply with these demands. When our ability to cope is pushed to the limit, bruxism may be nature's way of telling us to "slow down" and relax.

TEMPOROMANDIBULAR DISORDER

The temporomandibular joint is the hinge joint that connects the lower jaw to the upper jawbone. It functions through five pairs of muscles attached to the facial bones. The structures (bones, muscles, ligaments, and discs) that make it possible to open and close the mouth are very specialized and are required to work together to enable you to chew, speak, and swallow. The muscle pairs must work in proper balance so that stresses on both sides of the jaw are distributed as equally as possible. The temporomandibular joint is considered very complex because it is capable of making many different types of movements, including combinations of hinge and gliding actions. The juncture where the two joints are connected has a disc that acts like a shock absorber to biting and chewing forces. Any problem that prevents this complex system of structures from working together properly may result in cycles of pain, spasm (cramp), muscle tenderness, and damage to the tissue and joint. This is known as temporomandibular disorder (TMD).

Most researchers agree that temporomandibular disorders are grouped into three main categories, as follows. It is possible for a person to have one or more of these conditions at the same time.

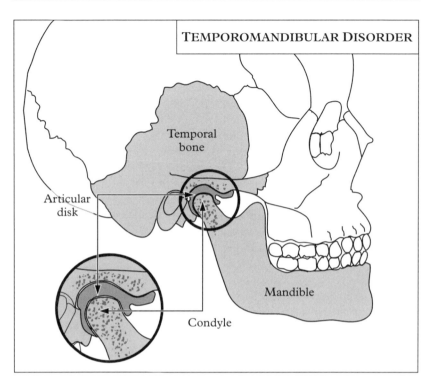

Figure 7

Myofascial pain is the most common form of TMD. It involves pain in the muscles that control the jaw function, the neck, and the shoulder.

Internal derangement of the joint means a dislocated jaw, a displaced disc, or injury to the condyle.

Degenerative joint disease includes osteoarthritis or rheumatoid arthritis in the jaw joint.

According to Dr. James Fricton, coordinator of the TMD and orofacial pain division at the University of Minnesota, "About 40 percent of Americans have some form of TMD, but only 5 percent to 10 percent have a problem that warrants treatment. Twice as many women as men have TMD, and it usually manifests itself in patients somewhere during the second to the fourth decade of life.

Symptoms that TMD sufferers have include:

◆ An ache in the area of the ear extending to the back of the head, into the face, neck, and shoulders
◆ Hearing a clicking or popping sound on opening and closing the mouth
◆ Pain brought on by yawning, opening the mouth widely, or chewing

184
▲

◆ Difficulty in opening the mouth and chewing (limited movement)
◆ Headaches that can mimic migraines, earaches, dizziness, and neck aches
◆ Jaws that "get stuck," lock, or "go out"
◆ Tenderness of the jaw muscles
◆ A sudden change in the way the upper and lower teeth fit together.

A combination of one or all of these symptoms can also be present for other problems. There are no exact causes and symptoms of TMD, so diagnosis can be difficult. After guidelines have been established it will be easier for health professionals to identify TMD correctly and make proper treatment choices for patients. It is important for your dentist to get a complete health/dental history in order to be able to make a diagnosis. Regular dental X rays and TMJ X rays (transcranial radiographs) are not useful in diagnosing this disorder. Diagnostic techniques that include *computerized tomography (CT scans), magnetic resonance imaging (MRI)* (pictures of the soft tissue), and *arthrography* (joint X rays using dye) are not usually needed unless the health professional strongly suspects arthritis or the pain and symptoms do not improve with treatment. It was reported in the September 1991 *Journal of the American Dental Association (JADA)* that the scientific literature does not support the use of jaw tracking, EMG, sonography, and thermography as diagnostic aids. "Guidelines have been proposed urging caution on their use because they are unable to provide any more information than a standard clinical examination." In addition, their reliability and validity remain unproven. The FDA reexamined this issue at a meeting in April 1995, and their recommendation is forthcoming.

Some clear-cut causes of TMD are arthritis, trauma, or severe stress. Unfortunately, TMD is usually a combination of factors, and not easily diagnosed. It is common for the disc in the temporomandibular joint to slip forward and click, pop, or even get stuck for a moment. In the absence of pain in the jaw this is a minor problem that does not require any treatment. Stress often results in clenching or grinding the teeth, which can be a factor that starts the cycle of muscle pain and spasms. Many researchers feel behavioral, psychological, and physical factors all contribute to TMD. It is important to note that at this time we do not know the exact causes of this disorder.

The treatment for TMD is quite variable. *The rule of thumb is least is best.* Conservative treatments do not invade the tissues of the face, jaw, or joint. Most temporomandibular joint disorders are temporary, and many times discomfort will eventually go away without treatment. Long-term studies have shown that 80 to 90 percent of patients can expect both good short-term results and little to no long-term problems after conservative therapy that reduces pain and restores normal function.

Conservative (reversible) treatments include counseling or biofeedback training to reduce emotional stress; muscle massage, relaxants, or tension monitors to aid in breaking the spasm-pain-spasm cycle; short-term soft diets to give the jaw muscles a chance to relax; using heat or ice packs; avoiding extreme jaw movements (e.g. yawning, gum chewing); physical therapy that focuses on gentle muscle stretching and relaxing exercises; and short-term use of anti-inflammatory and muscle relaxing drugs. Sometimes a plastic splint is recommended. Research studies suggest that flat-plane splints are initially more appropriate for TMD. Splints should only be used a short time (no more than three months), and should not cause any permanent changes to the bite.

Irreversible treatments for this disorder invade the tissue. They include injections into the muscle and joint; splints that change the bite; orthodontic treatment to bring the teeth into balanced occlusion; selectively grinding teeth to be sure they are in proper occlusion; and, at the extreme end, surgery might be necessary to correct a badly degenerated TMJ. Scientists have learned that irreversible treatments such as surgical replacement of jaw joints with artificial implants may cause severe pain and permanent jaw damage. Some of these devices do not function properly or may break apart over time in the jaw. *Before undergoing any surgery on the jaw joint, it is very important to get other independent opinions.* Pain clinics in hospitals and universities are a very good place to get advice and a second opinion. The current feeling of most scientists is that these replacements are of little value and may make the problem worse. A recent announcement from the National Institute of Dental Research states, "The Food and Drug Administration has recalled artificial jaw joint implants made by Vitek, Inc., which may break down and damage surrounding bone. If you have these implants, see your oral surgeon or dentist. If there are problems with your implants, the devices may need to be removed. Persons who have Vitek implants should call Medic Alert at 1-800-554-5297 for more information."

It takes time and patience to treat a long-term condition like TMD. Studies and recognition of TMD are relatively new to dentistry. The diagnosis is often made by process of elimination of other possible causes.

RESOURCE ORGANIZATIONS FOR TMD

The TMJ Association, Ltd.
6418 West Washington Boulevard
Wauwatosa, Wisconsin 53213
(414) 259-3223

TMJ Network
5 Corey Avenue
Shoneham, Massachusetts 02180
(617) 279-1146

U.S. Food and Drug Administration
Office of Consumer Affairs, HFE88
5600 Fishers Lane
Rockville, Maryland 20857
(301) 443-3170

National Oral Health Information Clearinghouse
1 NOHIC Way
Bethesda, Maryland 20892-3500
(301) 402-7364
(301) 907-8830 (fax)

13

Infectious Diseases

A recent report from the Center for Disease Control and Prevention (CDC) states the leading cause of death in the world today is infectious disease. This fact is linked primarily to the increase in human immunodeficiency virus (HIV) cases, the virus that causes acquired immunodeficiency syndrome (AIDS). Since 1981 there have been 14 million people, mainly from Africa and Asia, diagnosed with AIDS. Experts expect the number to reach 40 million by the year 2000. With all the publicity about AIDS, it is understandable to be concerned about contracting it at the dental office. However, the CDC says that the risk is extremely remote.

The development, implementation, and routine use of effective infection control in the dental office has required a major commitment by health professionals. Without question, the infection control protocol in today's dental practices differs by leaps and bounds from the protocol used in the 1980s. Attention regarding infection control was first noticed in the dental profession in the mid-1970s when an oral surgeon in California was implicated in the transmission of hepatitis B to a group of patients. Then, in July 1990, the issue of infection control in the dental office exploded when the Acer-Bergalis case became public. Ms. Bergalis claimed her dentist (Dr. Acer) transmitted AIDS to her. About the same time a survey in a popular dental trade magazine reported approximately 50 percent of the dental offices sterilized their hand pieces, and of those, only about 25 percent did so between each patient. Today 99 percent of the dentists in a recent survey indicated they sterilize their hand pieces. The dental offices of today have incorporated guidelines from both the Center for Disease Control and Prevention and the Occupational Safety and Health Administration (OSHA) into their patient treatment protocol, making dentistry safer today than it ever has been. These guidelines advocate the use of *universal precautions*, which are designed to protect the health professionals, the staff, and the patients from contracting all blood-borne pathogens. This includes HIV and hepatitis B.

HIV

AIDS is caused by the retrovirus known as human immunodeficiency virus (HIV) type 1. It is transmitted by sex (semen, vaginal fluids), blood or blood products, or an infected mother to the fetus or newborn at birth. Infection with HIV usually results in a disease associated with progressive immune dysregulation, dysfunction, and deficiency (e.g. AIDS). Individuals with the virus can remain asymptomatic for many years. It usually takes about 10 years after the initial infection before the first signs of AIDS appear.

The May 1995 *Annals of Internal Medicine* reports in a study that after looking at a group of health care workers with AIDS it found there is no evidence of doctor-to-patient transmission of the AIDS virus. CDC scientists say they will never be able to explain the Acer case. However, researchers agree "if HIV were easily transmitted from health care workers to patients evidence of such transmissions would have been detected in these investigations."

The virus that causes AIDS is readily destroyed by disinfection and sterilization measures that dentists routinely use to control the transmission of all infectious diseases. To protect the health of the dentist, his staff, and his patients dentists have implemented universal precautions. This means they treat each patient with the same protective measures to prevent the transmission of the virus that causes AIDS or any other infectious disease. The ADA has taken the position that the guidelines are now part of acceptable standard of care to be followed by all dentists. Any health professional who does not follow these precautions is liable for a considerable fine from OSHA, whose representatives make surprise visits to offices. Universal precautions for infection control include:

1. Wearing masks, gloves, and protective eyewear and garments
2. Sterilizing dental instruments and hand pieces (drills) after each use
3. Washing hands before and after each treatment
4. Changing gloves after each patient
5. Cleaning and disinfecting the surfaces in the treatment room and equipment after each patient
6. Disposing of needles and other sharp items in special puncture-proof containers

7. Disposing of waste items and contaminated material properly.

When you go to the dentist for treatment, you can visibly observe if the dentist and his staff are wearing gloves, protective garments, and masks. Notice while you are in the office if surfaces and equipment seem clean and neat. Since precautions that involve sterilization and disinfection are completed before you enter the treatment room ask the dentist or a staff member if hand pieces and all instruments are being heat sterilized between each patient.

Dental offices use various acceptable methods to sterilize and disinfect in order to kill bacteria and viruses. It is best to sterilize, as opposed to disinfect, as many items as possible. A good rule of thumb is to sterilize all instruments, including the hand pieces, and to disinfect all surface areas in the treatment room. The CDC and the American Dental Association guidelines recommend heat sterilization of all critical and semicritical instruments. Critical instruments are those that touch bone or penetrate soft tissue. Semicritical instruments are those that come in contact with mucous membranes, but do not penetrate bone or soft tissue. For semicritical instruments that cannot withstand heat processing it is acceptable to use high-level chemical disinfection with a tuberculocidal EPA-registered agent. Proper sterilization involves first cleaning the debris off the items to be sterilized. Then the items are usually placed in an ultrasonic cleaner. Next the items are rinsed, put in sterilization pouches, and placed in the autoclave for sterilization. Acceptable methods for autoclaving include steam under pressure, dry heat in an ovenlike environment, and chemical vapor sterilization.

Disinfection procedures are used on surface areas and equipment that cannot be removed for cleaning and sterilization. These include countertops, handles to drawers and the light at the chair, X-ray unit heads, and the chair and dental unit. Disinfection of these surfaces should be done between each patient to assure that the operatory is clean before any new patients start treatment.

Any items that cannot be sterilized such as masks, paper drapes, gloves, etc. are made with the intent they will only be used once and then disposed of properly.

Some discussion has been circulated about mandating that health care workers be tested for HIV. This sounds like an easy solution. However, since only a positive test result has any significance this would not protect the patient. The AIDS test relies on the presence of antibodies that can take six months or longer to develop after the person is infected. Therefore, a negative test does not provide assurance that a person does not have the AIDS virus. Experts all agree the best way to deal with the AIDS virus, or any other infectious disease, is to use proper preventive measures and ongoing public education.

You should address any concerns about universal precautions to your dentist or his staff. They should be very willing to answer your concerns.

The ADA has cautioned all health professionals that the Americans with Disabilities Act (AwDA) prohibits discrimination against people with disabilities in public places, such as the dental office. Patients diagnosed with both HIV and AIDS are considered disabled by the act. The ADA has supported the policy of not refusing treatment to patients with HIV or AIDS as long as the patient's dental condition is within their realm of competence. If not, dentists may refer the patient to a specialist for treatment. The ADA has taken the position that as long as universal precautions are followed the chances of transmitting the disease are very remote. Anyone refusing treatment to these individuals solely based on the fact they have AIDS or HIV is subject to legal action.

TUBERCULOSIS

The *New England Journal of Medicine* recently reported a study that details a single untreated man with active TB who infected 41 patrons of a Minneapolis bar. Tuberculosis is caused by the bacterium *M. tuberculosis*. It is spread by airborne particles, known as droplet nuclei, that are generated into the air when people with TB sneeze, cough, or speak. The particles generated are so small they can stay airborne for prolonged periods and spread throughout a building. This infectious disease has been on the upswing in recent years. From 1955 to 1985 tuberculosis was in decline in this country. Then with the increase in susceptibility of AIDS patients to TB, an increase in immigrants coming into this country with TB, a decrease in health care resources directed at TB control, and the increased crowding of prisons, shelters, and nursing homes, the incidence of the disease has increased. *USA Today* recently reported the 1993 budget for TB control in New York City was $40 million, up from $4 million in 1988. The cost of the resurgence of TB is predicted to easily exceed $1 billion in that city alone. A recent survey shows there are an estimated 10 to 15 million people in the United States infected with TB. Approximately 1,500 people died of TB in 1995.

In October 1994 the CDC announced guidelines for preventing the transmission of tuberculosis in health care settings. OSHA is expected to soon be releasing their guidelines for protecting workers from occupational exposure to TB. These guidelines are expected to be very similar to the CDC guidelines.

The CDC divides health care facilities into five levels of risk—minimal, very low, low, intermediate, and high. Most dental offices fall into the minimal or very low level of risk. A minimal level of risk dental office is one that does not treat patients with TB, and no TB cases were reported in the community during the preceding year. A very low risk dental office does not treat TB patients, but there have been TB cases reported in the community during the preceding year.

The CDC guidelines state "the symptoms for which patients seek treatment in a dental care setting are not likely to be caused by infectious TB. Unless a patient requiring dental care coincidentally has TB, it is unlikely that infectious TB will be encountered in the dental setting. Furthermore, the generation of droplet nuclei containing *M. tuberculosis* during dental procedures has not been demonstrated. Therefore, the risk of transmission in most dental settings is probably quite low."

The CDC requires dental offices to develop a written infection control protocol for screening patients with active TB and referring suspected TB patients to appropriate facilities for assessment and/or treatment. Most offices screen patients for TB when they take the patient's health history. CDC guidelines state dentists should defer elective and emergency dental care for both suspected and active TB to appropriate facilities. The CDC feels typical dental offices cannot safely treat infectious TB patients. This is important because TB is considered a disability under the AwDA, just as AIDS and HIV are disabilities. The reason dentists are not required to treat active TB patients is because the threat to the health and safety of others cannot be reduced to an acceptable level by reasonable accommodation. However, once the patient is rendered noninfectious he can return to the dentist for treatment. If no complications exist, patients can be rendered noninfectious in two to three weeks. With AIDS patients, the use of universal precautions renders them noninfectious so they can be treated in the dental office without threat to the safety of others.

The CDC also requires dental offices to have written protocols for handling patients who are in the office and suspected of having TB. They should be given facial tissues so they can cover their nose and mouth when coughing or sneezing.

In addition, the CDC requires dental offices to have initial baseline TB screening for employees when they are hired.

HEPATITIS B

Most researchers agree it is much more likely that hepatitis B will be transmitted in the dental office than HIV. It is transmitted by blood and blood products, it is mainly associated with liver disease. In 1992, OSHA, with the endorsement of the ADA, mandated the dentist to make this vaccine series available to all employees at the dentist's expense. The vaccine usually costs about $70 per injection, and it is necessary to have three injections over a period of time. OSHA considers part-time, temporary, and probationary workers as employees. The guidelines allow newly hired employees to participate in patient care during the two-to-six-month period it takes to complete the series of vaccine injections. Within ten days of employment all employees are required to receive training in how to properly handle blood-borne pathogens. If an employee declines to have the vaccine a document to that effect must be signed and kept in the OSHA recordkeeping manual. The vaccine is about 90 percent effective.

MOUTH SORES

Mouth sores, which can occur either inside the mouth or outside around the mouth on the lips, affect 20 to 40 percent of the population. They can significantly hinder eating and speaking, which leads to anorexia and a poor quality of life. Accurate diagnosis is essential for appropriate treatment. Painful ulcers inside the mouth are called canker sores. These can occur singly or in clusters, and they may last from 10 to 14 days. For whatever reason, women have these more frequently than men. There is no consensus of opinion why these occur. Several sources tell us that these may result as a "localized immune reaction." Deficiencies in iron, vitamin B-12, and folic acid seem to increase susceptibility. Stress and local trauma are the most common precipitating factors.

If these reoccur in an individual they are called *recurrent aphthous ulcers*. Reoccurence usually comes on two to three times a year. It is interesting to note that at least one study to date has indicated that some patients prone to aphthous ulcers report a significant decrease in ulcerations when the foaming agent (sodium lauryl sulfate) found in many toothpastes is removed. Relief can occur by using a topical anesthetic mouthwash such as 2 percent lidocaine before meals, or by applying Orabase paste on the ulcers four times/day. The FDA has recently approved an aloe vera derivative (acemannan hydrogel) that has been found very effective in treating oral ulcers. It accelerates healing and reduces pain associated with aphthous ulcers. In contrast to other medications for this problem, acemannan hydrogel does not have the disagreeable taste and texture of traditional therapies. It also does not sting when applied. The research for this product was done at Baylor College of Dentistry in Dallas. It will be marketed under the name

Carrasyn Oral Wound Dressing by Carrington Laboratories. Dr. T. Rees said in a Baylor news release, "We currently are investigating this as a possible method of treating any irritated area in the mouth, from whatever source, whether from a compromised immune system or physical trauma."

When mouth sores occur outside the mouth on the lips, they are usually caused by the infamous *herpes simplex* virus. They are common in infants and young children, but may also occur in teenagers and adults. These mouth sores are frequently referred to as *fever blisters* or *cold sores*. They can be brought about by mild trauma as from a dental appointment, sunburn, systemic illness, immunosuppressive therapy, cancer chemotherapy, or food allergies. These have also been associated with anxiety or, in some cases, the onset of a woman's menstrual cycle. The usual course of these bothersome sores is seven to ten days. In cases of *recurrent herpes labialis* the patient experiences a sensation of fullness, burning, and itching before the vesicle develops. The lesions need not be confined to the lips, but can be found extending to the roof of the mouth, the hard palate, and the associated gum tissue (gingiva). If there is direct contact with these lesions through kissing, eating, or drinking they can be transmitted to another individual. There are several tests available for detecting herpes simplex in oral lesions, but researchers feel the most reliable is a viral culture with immunotyping of the isolates. However, it takes several days to get the results. Some relief occurs in these lesions when a mouth rinse of either 2 percent lidocaine is used before meals or a half teaspoon of sodium bicarbonate mouthwash in 8 ounces of water is used as needed. Your dentist can prescribe a topical application of the antiviral agent Vidarabine or Acyclovir to aid in limiting the spread of these mouth sores. Ice on the lesions helps reduce swelling and petroleum jelly helps prevent bleeding or cracking of these sores. Taking Acyclovir tablets for 10 days (five times/day) has been shown to give relief in severe cases. There is no real cure. Do not put alcohol on these sores. This only invites the creation of resistant strains. Also, do not put an anticortisteroid on these sores because this will spread the virus.

ORAL FUNGAL INFECTIONS

Oral candidiasis (thrush) is one of the most common pathological conditions affecting the oral mucosa (inside of the mouth). It appears as a smooth, creamy white or yellow plaque on any mucosal surface. When the plaque is wiped away the underlying mucosa is red. The infections are usually localized. Oral candidiasis is associated with a decreased host defense caused by a variety of different drug therapies (broad-spectrum antibiotics), systemic diseases (diabetis mellitus, cancer), and local changes in the oral cavity (radiation to the head and neck, Sjogren's syndrome, inflammation under a denture). All of these are associated with decreased salivary flow, which is the underlying cause of oral candidiasis. It is important for health professionals to recognize oral fungal infections and make sure the cause is determined because they are markers for early signs of immune deterioration (HIV). The most common medications prescribed to treat oral candidiasis are Nystatin oral lozenges and rinse and Clotrimazole oral lozenges and suspension.

14

Dental-Related Pain

Many times dental-related pain is difficult to diagnose. Most commonly, these patients are referred to endodontists, oral and maxillofacial surgeons, or periodontists. Since there is no approved ADA specialty program to handle this type of problem, patients have difficulty knowing where to go to get help. Many authorities feel the best place to seek help is at a chronic pain clinic that is associated with a large medical center that includes a dental school. Usually these clinics have dentists on staff who are familiar with these types of cases. These clinics have access to dental specialists in all areas of dentistry, so it is possible to get a multidisciplinary approach to help resolve the problem. It is generally accepted among authorities that a conservative and reversible approach to treatment is always better. Several types of dental related pain are discussed below.

CHRONIC FACIAL PAIN

Chronic facial pain is a problem that affects a patient's quality of life significantly because it interferes with their ability to function at home, work, or in a social setting. The gravity of this problem presents a tremendous challenge to health professionals in their attempts to investigate and treat this disorder. The average patient with this problem seeks care from four to six clinicians and spends thousands of dollars in search of relief. It is not surprising that patients seek so many different health professionals for treatment when you consider the confusion among dentists and physicians as to exactly what constitutes chronic facial pain and how it should be treated. Unfortunately, this has resulted in leaving many patients with irreversible damage and even more pain, which has contributed to a growing number of malpractice cases. In general, the problem lies in the fact that many clinicians are trying to manage problems that are beyond their expertise.

Most of the literature on this subject has been derived from clinical data instead of from a research basis. As a result, many currently accepted theories for treatment exist without the benefit of research that employs well-defined control groups, minimal bias, and the use of appropriate statistical methods. At this time there are no standardized diagnostic criteria for researchers to use to compare results. Thus, progress in improving therapy has been hindered by the acceptance of treatments and theories that lack scientific basis. Too many times, complicated, unnecessary, and expensive treatments are used when more conservative treatment would achieve similar or even better results.

Most authorities agree the most effective approach to treating chronic facial pain of muscle origin seems to be multidisciplinary. The focus should be on identifying all possible contributing factors and managing them by using physical, dental, and behavioral therapies. At this time, most authorities are in agreement that *all therapies should be reversible and conservative. Irreversible therapy is seldom recommended.*

The complexity of the head and neck and the potential for numerous pathological conditions that can cause pain makes it mandatory for the health provider to consider carefully all possible answers to the patient's problem. Clinicians should begin by taking a detailed medical/dental history and a physical examination to rule out any medical disorders (systemic diseases that manifest in the head). If the results are negative, the next step is to rule out any dental problems (e.g. filling or root canal therapy needed, periodontal disease, etc.) that could be causing the pain. If these results are negative, then the clinician should examine the temporomandibular joint, keeping in mind that joint "clicking noises do not necessarily eliminate other structures as the cause of symptoms. A diagnosis of masticatory pain can only be considered after all other options have been exhausted. Muscle splinting is an appropriate diagnosis if pain begins from the date of a placement of a restoration or a prosthesis (i.e. full or partial denture). Acute myositis is considered if there has been a recent trauma to the face, as long as infection, a systemic disease, or a jaw fracture have been ruled out as the problem. When pain has been present more than a month, a tentative diagnosis of myofascial pain or masticatory myalgia may be appropriate.

Chronic pain can be treated with several reversible procedures: physical therapy (including massage), ultrasound, accupressure, application of moist heat or ice to the area, prescribing anti-inflammatory agents, electrical (electrogalvanic) stimulation, active and passive exer-

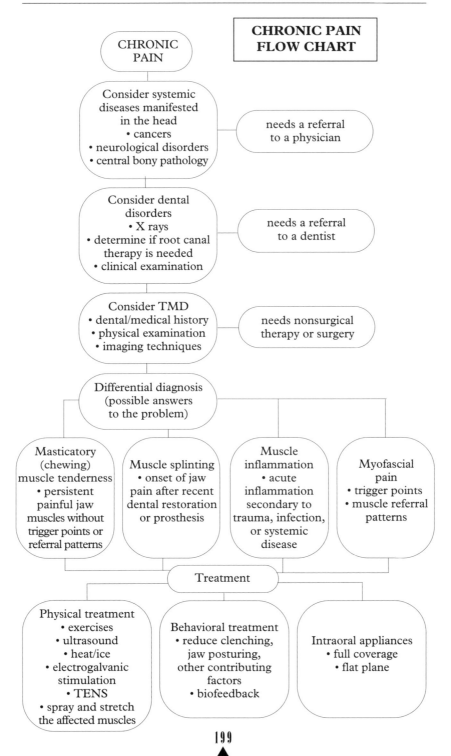

CHRONIC PAIN FLOW CHART

CHRONIC PAIN

Consider systemic diseases manifested in the head
• cancers
• neurological disorders
• central bony pathology

→ needs a referral to a physician

Consider dental disorders
• X rays
• determine if root canal therapy is needed
• clinical examination

→ needs a referral to a dentist

Consider TMD
• dental/medical history
• physical examination
• imaging techniques

→ needs nonsurgical therapy or surgery

Differential diagnosis (possible answers to the problem)

Masticatory (chewing) muscle tenderness
• persistent painful jaw muscles without trigger points or referral patterns

Muscle splinting
• onset of jaw pain after recent dental restoration or prosthesis

Muscle inflammation
• acute inflammation secondary to trauma, infection, or systemic disease

Myofascial pain
• trigger points
• muscle referral patterns

Treatment

Physical treatment
• exercises
• ultrasound
• heat/ice
• electrogalvanic stimulation
• TENS
• spray and stretch the affected muscles

Behavioral treatment
• reduce clenching, jaw posturing, other contributing factors
• biofeedback

Intraoral appliances
• full coverage
• flat plane

cises of the affected area, spraying with an aerosol skin coolant in combination with stretch techniques to treat trigger points, transcutaneous electrical nerve stimulation (TENS), and biofeedback. The most common treatment for chronic facial pain is a flat plane splint that covers the entire arch.

It is a well-accepted fact that the diagnosis of chronic facial pain is difficult, and once it has been diagnosed it is always best to take the conservative, reversible approach to treatment.

MYOFASCIAL PAIN

Myofascial pain (MFP) is a regional, dull muscular ache characterized by localized tender spots known as "trigger points" in the involved muscle and its associated area. It can be localized to one muscle group, such as the chewing muscles, or have a more generalized distribution throughout the body. It is necessary for health professionals to palpate (massage) the affected muscle area to duplicate the patient's pain before a diagnosis can be made. It must be noted that some people who do not have the symptoms of MFP report pain during muscle palpation, so a diagnosis of MFP cannot be made for these otherwise asymptomatic patients. Another consideration is that there are many other disorders that can cause secondary muscle pain, so these must be ruled out before the patient is treated for MFP.

Dentists usually prescribe flat-plane acrylic splints for MFP. Alternative therapies may be used to increase the effects of the splint therapy. These include:

◆ acupuncture
◆ biofeedback
◆ heat and cold applications
◆ jaw exercises
◆ massage
◆ relaxation therapy
◆ self-management
◆ stress management
◆ trigger point injections
◆ trigger point compression

When considering all of the above, the therapies presumed to be the most effective alternative methods of treatment are acupuncture, biofeedback, relaxation therapy, and stress management.

Self-management is a standard treatment for MFP. Studies show 60 to 90 percent of the patients report improvement in their symptoms when using self-management exclusively. Self-management treatment includes limiting the activity of the chewing muscles (eat soft food; don't yawn or chew gum), eliminating parafunctional habits (e.g. clenching), applying heat and cold to the affected areas, eliminating caffeine, and using over-the-counter anti-inflammatory medications. Prescription anti-inflammatory medications, muscle relaxants, and low-dose antidepressants are often used as adjunctive therapy for patients with MFP.

Currently there is no scientifically determined protocol or consensus of opinion among authorities for treating patients with MFP. When a patient does not respond to self-management, an evaluation by a dentist, physical therapist, and a psychologist is appropriate to determine which intervention or combination of interventions is appropriate.

ATYPICAL FACE PAIN

Atypical face pain (AFP) is a condition that often responds poorly to most accepted therapies. However, a high percentage of these patients take multiple medications for the problem daily. Virtually all authorities agree the most common cause of this problem is depression and anxiety, and it has a psychological etiology (origin). Usually the condition is diagnosed by a psychiatrist. AFP patients consistently experience tenderness in the upper jaw area next to the root ends of the molars. Patients with this condition usually have an elevated temperature in the affected area. This condition may be confused with temporomandibular disorder. However, patients with TMD usually have intermittent symptoms that relate to the function of their jaw. AFP usually is identified on the basis of exclusion, as the symptoms don't fit any other diagnostic category.

BURNING MOUTH SYNDROME

Burning mouth syndrome (BMS) is characterized by a constant pain in the mouth with no apparent lesions. The pain is usually on both sides of the mouth and involves multiple sites. The regions involved, in decreasing frequency, are the front part of the tongue, front portion of the roof of the mouth, and the inside of the lower lip. The pain is usually of moderate to severe intensity, and is often described as burning, tender, and annoying. It affects more than 1 million U.S. adults, and it usually occurs in post-menopausal females. Studies show there is a lower prevalence of BMS in the U.S. than in Canada. Even though the pain and burning associated with BMS is found in the mouth and lip area physicians are more likely than dentists to treat these patients. BMS has been associated with numerous oral and systemic conditions. The symptoms are dry mouth, oral burning, persistent altered taste perception, thirst, irritability, depression, changes in eating habits, and a decreased desire to socialize. The symptoms stop without predictability, with spontaneous remission of symptoms occuring in some patients. It is often necessary to get input from several health care providers in different disciplines. Many times the symptoms do not respond to medication.

Most authorities feel the cause of BMS is either an oral disorder or a sytemic condition. Oral disorders associated with this condition include:

- candidiasis
- allergies to dental acrylic
- dentures that do not fit properly
- parafunctional habits
- periodontal disease
- peripheral nerve damage
- salivary gland dysfunction
- taste dysfunction
- noninflammatory tongue with discolorations
- viral infections
- mouth ulcers

Most studies have reported there is no consistent prevalence of any specific medical condition linked to BMS. It has been reported, however, that there is a higher occurrence of many health complaints, medication usage, and chronic pain conditions in BMS patients. Systemic causes of BMS include:

- anemia
- central nervous system disorders
- diabetes
- hematological disorders
- nutritional disorders
- psychiatric and psychological disorders (mood changes)
- Sjogren's syndrome (characterized by dry eyes and mouth)

Other possible causes include menopause, food and drug allergies, smoking, spices (specifically cinnamon), and medications. A suggested anecdotal remedy has been the use of chilled apple-juice rinses to relieve the symptoms.

BMS is a common but poorly understood oralfacial pain disorder that is difficult to diagnose and to manage. Many feel standardized symptom and diagnostic criteria should be formulated so other disciplines can identify effective and reliable treatment strategies.

PHANTOM TOOTH PAIN

Phantom tooth pain (PTP) is a condition of chronic dental pain for no discernible pathological reason. It is a phenomenon that occurs in teeth after successful endodontic treatment and in extraction sites. A correlation in medicine would be pain in a phantom limb after it has been amputated. Adults (both male and female) in any age group are susceptible, but there are currently no reported cases in children. Patients are considered candidates for PTP if they meet the following criteria:

◆ continued chronic tooth pain after successful dental treatment or extraction of the tooth
◆ clinical examination and X-ray findings are normal
◆ findings do not suggest any other medical problems in the head and neck area
◆ patients fail to respond to therapies that normally alleviate dental pain (narcotics, extractions)

It is necessary to have normal findings from comprehensive clinical, neurologic, and radiographic assessments before PTP can be considered as a diagnosis. The pain associated with PTP is widely regarded as psychogenic.

15

Dental Insurance: What You'd Better Know

Spending for dental services rose from $27.1 billion in 1985 to over $42 billion in 1994. The Health Care Financing Administration (HCFA) projects that these figures will reach $90 billion by the year 2000.

Today, approximately half of the population in the United States (between 113 million and 125 million Americans) is covered by private dental insurance companies. Compare this to the figures in 1970, when there were only 12 million dental insurance policyholders. According to the ADA Survey of Dental Practice over 63 percent of the patients who visit the dentist have a private dental insurance program. However, about 53 percent of all dental costs are paid out-of-pocket by private patients. Dental plans are popular benefits among employers because their moderate costs are under control. In 1990, while medical plans rose about 25 percent from the previous year, dental plans only rose about 6 percent. This trend continues today. One reason for the low cost of dental coverage is the moderate claims experience of this industry and the strictly defined benefits. Dentistry has always been preventive oriented, thus reducing the need for expenditures for more expensive procedures. Managed care plans are easy to sell to employers because they perceive they will be receiving certain services "free" for a very low premium cost.

The chances are that your dental insurance is a benefit to you from either your place of employment or your trade union. Look closely at your policy because all dental insurance coverage is not the same.

There are four levels of coverage that dental insurance policies offer: diagnostic and preventive (examinations, X rays, tooth cleaning, and fluoride application to the teeth), basic (restorations, endodontics, and routine extractions), major (dentures, crown and bridge procedures), and orthodontics. When dental plans are marketed, they are priced according to which of these four levels of coverage will be included in the plan. The least expensive plans include only preventive care. More expensive plans have preventive and basic care. The most expensive plans have all four levels of coverage. Orthodontic coverage is a major service in terms of expense, but it is categorized separately.

Dental benefits are organized into three categories: indemnity, managed care, and employer based self-insurance.

INDEMNITY PLANS

Indemnity dental insurance, also known as *traditional* or *fee for service* insurance, is a contract between the insured and the insurance company. A premium is paid by the insurer (employer and/or employee) to the insurance company, and in return specific benefits are paid to the insurer when a claim is received for covered procedures performed by the dentist or his staff. Usually, these plans pay 100 percent for preventive care, 80 percent for basic care, and 50 percent for major care. The insurance company assumes the risk that the total claims paid out will not exceed the total premiums collected, thus generating a profit. If your dentist's fee exceeds the plan's maximum allowance it does not mean your dentist has overcharged for the procedure. The dentist does not have any control over these allowances. Insurance companies set these maximum allowances with the idea in mind that they will not have to pay out more for claims than they will receive in premiums in any given year. They are in business to make money. Therefore, the maximum allowance is an arbitrary number that they use to insure a profit at the end of the year.

Claims are paid by insurance companies from three basic formats. *Unscheduled plans* pay benefits based on a percentile for the prevailing fees in a geographic area. *Scheduled plans* pay benefits based on a percentage of a fee schedule that is set by the insurance company, also called a *usual and customary rate (UCR)*. The insurance company, not the dentists in the area, determines the UCR by utilizing a wide variety of methods. Because there is a lack of government regulations on determining UCRs, patients should ask the insurance representatives how they are determined before they purchase the plan. It is also important to know how often the data is updated. Payments for *direct reimbursement plan* levels of coverage are based on the amount of dental expenditure in a plan year instead of categories of treatment. These plans usually pay on the following schedule:

100 percent of the first $100
80 percent of the next $500
50 percent of the next $2,000

The annual maximum is usually $1,500 per person enrolled in the plan. This type of plan is very flexible because it allows enrollees to obtain coverage for whatever treatment is needed from the dentist of their choice.

MANAGED CARE

The three basic managed care plans are as follows: *managed fee-for-service plans, health maintenance organizations (HMOs),* and *preferred provider organizations (PPOs).* Managed care plans use a variety of delivery systems to control the cost and quality of dental care. With these plans patients are not required to complete claim forms, and they do not pay deductibles or copayments for basic and preventive services they receive from their general dentist. In recent years it has been the trend for insurance companies to phase out traditional indemnity plans (based on fee-for-service and UCR) and transfer their financial risk to the provider by promoting managed care plans. Initially, these plans are popular with patients, but ultimately they prove to be much less desirable than expected.

Before purchasing a managed care plan you should consider:

1. What is the dentist/patient ratio on the plan?
2. Where are the contracted dentists geographically located?
3. Does the plan provide for specialty referrals?
4. What is the enrollee's copayment for procedures completed at the general dentist's office? What is the copayment for procedures referred to the specialist? Usually when it is necessary for a specialist to complete a procedure, the copayment is more than when the assigned general dentist completes the same procedure. The reason is the specialist does not usually receive a capitation check each month from the carrier to offset his expenses.

5. What provisions are made for emergency treatment both at home and away from home?
6. What is the average waiting period for an initial appointment and between appointments?
7. What criteria is used for selecting the general dentists and specialists on the plan?

Managed Fee-for-service

Managed fee-for-service plans pay the dentist for treatment on a fee-for-service basis. However, the dentist must agree to certain contractual management provisions in order to be eligible for direct payment. The maximum table of allowances for fees on these plans is lower than the usual and customary allowance used in traditional fee-for-service plans. Usually the patient has a copayment for basic and major services.

HMOs

According to Interstudy (a Minnesota-based research organization), health maintenance organization enrollment in 1993 increased 11.6 percent to 45 million people. This is way up from 30 million in 1987. Given this trend, managed care plans are projected to capture 20 to 40 percent of the dental insurance market by the year 2000. These plans are typically less expensive to the enrollee because the reimbursement is fixed. Another advantage of these plans is the review systems that are used to evaluate the offices that are included. Usually a representative comes to the facility or office on an annual basis to evaluate the credentials of the dentist, and the physical aspects and recordkeeping practices of the office. One disadvantage of these plans is a limited provider network. Also, the schedule of services provided on the plan is usually more limited than in some of the other types of programs. Another disadvantage of these plans is the difficulty of getting patients transferred from one office to another due to the loss of a provider or a desire on the patient's part to change providers. Statistics reflect that most capitation programs are seriously underfunded for what they promise to deliver.

HMOs can be organized in two ways. A dental HMO facility can pay dentists a salary to work in the facility treating patients enrolled in the program. Treatment guidelines are set by the facility and guided by a corporate philosophy. These guidelines must be followed by the dentist, even if they conflict with the dentist's personal philosophy. The facility assumes all the financial risk. The cost for the patient to belong to the program is fixed, regardless of the treatment needed. The premium, which can only be increased when the policy is renewed, is based on the number of people in the immediate family who are eligible for benefits. Usually patients do not see the same dentist each time they come for treatment. Problems sometimes occur in these facilities when the patient load becomes too large for the dentists to handle. The result is that dental care is not always attended to quickly. This HMO concept is good for families who cannot otherwise afford dental care or for elderly on a fixed income.

The other HMO model, also known as an Independent Practice Association (IPA), involves contracting a group of independent dentists in private practice to provide a risk pool from which specific services to eligible patients can be provided for a monthly capitation payment ($8–$10) each month for each person enrolled in the plan assigned to their office. The enrollees are assigned to one of the participating dentists. The monthly capitation payment is made without concern for the number of services rendered or the beneficiaries treated. In return, the IPA markets the plan to patient groups. With this plan, the dentist assumes all the financial risk. The cost to the patient for this program is fixed (based on the number of family members utilizing the program), regardless of treatment needed. In order to make a profit the capitation payments to the dentist must exceed the cost of rendering a promised package of dental benefits to the enrollees. This encourages the dentist to try to keep patient utilization of benefits to a minimum. If a specialist is needed, the general dentist is the "gatekeeper" who must make the referral. In some plans payment to the contracted specialist must come from the capitation funds paid to the general dentist. This can discourage the general dentist from making necessary referrals. In other capitation plans, the specialist agrees to provide services at a discounted fee that is paid by the enrollee directly to the specialist. This arrangement is more conducive for general dentists to make sure patients get referral care when it is necessary. Recently some capitation plans have begun to ask the patient to pay a small copayment each time they visit the dentist's office. This has encouraged more dentists to participate in the plan, which is a benefit to the patients. When a plan does not have enough dentists participating in it, patients begin to have long delays between appointments and trouble getting in to see their assigned dentist when they have an emergency situation.

PPOs

A *preferred provider organization* (PPO), also known as a *contract dental organization* (CDO), enrolls general dentists and specialists in private practice who contractually agree to provide services to eligible patients for the plan's fee schedule or for discounts from their current fees. Patients can go outside the "network" of dentists, but the benefits paid will be reduced and the plan's fee schedule will not be binding to dentists not contracted on the plan. The dentists are paid on a fee-for-service basis; therefore, the dentist is generally not at financial risk. One disadvantage of a PPO is that utilization often increases because the fees are discounted. This forces the dentist to have to render more services in order to make the same income, causing the dentist-patient relationship to suffer because the dentist has less time available to spend with each patient. This also makes it more difficult to get an appointment for treatment. An advantage of the PPO to the dentist is that the plan increases his patient pool because it refers enrollees to his practice. A disadvantage is the dentist's loss of control of the fees and contractual agreements for management of the practice (e.g. quality assurance, utilization reviews, and audits). Patients considering this plan should consider what criteria the insurance company uses when selecting dentists as providers on this plan.

SELF-INSURANCE

Self-insurance by the employer can either be *direct reimbursement* (DR) or *administrative services only* (ASO). With DR the employee pays the dentist when treatment is rendered and receives reimbursement for all or part of that payment from the employer. Employers can either self-administer the plan or hire an outside administrator. ASO plans provide the employer with a review of the claims, utilization review, review of the fees, and claims administration. The employer pays the claims after the ASO review. The dissatisfaction of many enrollees with managed care plans has caused an increasing number of employers to offer self-insurance plans in their benefit packages.

Most dental insurance plans involve some form of copayment, deductible, and maximum benefit. The bottom line is that you are responsible for some part of the payment. If you are familiar with insurance terminology, you'll have a clearer idea of exactly what your coverage entails. The following are some common terms used by insurance companies in their policies:

carrier This is another term for the dental insurance company that offers dental insurance benefits to eligible members of the plan.

coordination of benefits Utilizing the benefits of both spouses' plans for all members of the family when their coverage includes themselves, their spouse, and dependent children in their family.

copayment   A portion of the dental fee is paid by the patient. Often diagnostic and preventive services are excluded from copayment requirements in a policy to encourage regular dental care. The amount of the copayment can vary. Most indemnity plans have a 20 percent copayment and reimburse at 80 percent of their UCR. Managed care plans often have a flat-fee copayment for specific procedures. It should be noted that several state attorney generals' opinions have determined that waiver of a copayment by the dentist is illegal. The fee charged the patient must be the same as the fee charged to the insurance company.

deductible   An initial amount that the patient is liable for at the beginning of each fiscal/calendar year for each insured person (usually up to two to three per family) before the person becomes eligible for plan benefits.

dependent   The spouse or child of a subscriber to a dental health plan who is eligible for dental benefits.

exclusions   Procedures not covered under the plan.

explanation of benefits (EOB)   A form generated by an insurance company that is sent to the enrollee and the providing dentist that explains both payment of benefits and denials of coverage. This form needs to be attached to claims sent to a secondary insurance company so they can coordinate benefits.

plan maximum   The maximum amount the plan will pay for dental care in a fiscal/calendar year for each eligible person. Usually a plan maximum is between $500 and $1,500. Many plans also have a maximum lifetime benefit for each plan enrollee.

predetermination (also called **preauthorization**)   The amount the insurance company will allow for a procedure as determined prior to treatment. To get predetermination, your dentist must submit his proposed treatment and X rays to the insurance company. With the aid of consultants, the insurer will determine the benefit coverage that will be reimbursed for each procedure after treatment is completed. Some carriers request that all claims over a set amount (usually $100 to $300) be preauthorized, unless the patient needs immediate treatment to relieve pain.

provider   The dentist who is providing the dental treatment.

subscriber   The person who is eligible for dental insurance coverage. Most subscribers receive dental insurance benefits at their place of employment.

table of allowances   As the name implies, this is the maximum dollar benefit for each specific dental procedure, regardless of the fee charged. As you might expect, these tables seldom keep pace with the inflation rate.

usual and customary (UC)   A percentage of a dental fee paid by an insurer based upon an average fee for that specific service in the geographic area in which the service is performed. Geographic areas are usually divided according to ZIP codes. Sometimes, however, the insurer determines the UCR by taking the average fee charged for a procedure over a wide region (several adjacent states).

Mastery of dental insurance vocabulary will make you a better consumer. When you have questions about your coverage, it is best to contact your insurance company directly. Many dental offices are very knowledgeable about the many plans in their area, but there are so many that the only sure way to have correct information is to go to the source, the insurance company. When looking at your coverage always keep in mind that the predetermined amount for a specific procedure will only be paid within the ceiling set by the plan maximum. If there is a discrepancy between the two, the plan maximum takes precedence.

The important thing to realize is that each dental policy is unique. For example, some policies have a waiting period after enrollment before coverage actually begins. Policies may also have a clause that extends coverage completed within three months after coverage ends so long as the treatment began while the coverage was still in effect. Some plans also offer *COBRA* plans to enrollees at the time of termination of employment. These plans allow enrollees to have limited coverage for a premium that is usually much more expensive. The possibilities are endless. Basically, when an employer begins negotiations with an insurance carrier the extent of coverage in the policy is based entirely on how much the employer wants to set aside in the budget for this benefit. The insurance carrier uses factors such as the age, job description, and past claim experience for this group and similar groups to determine the cost per person for coverage. And the employer takes the needs of the group to be covered into consideration. For example, a policy for a group of young, newly married people would probably include more items related to children than a policy for an older group.

Subscribers should be aware that some dental insurance carriers are beginning to take a "new approach" to dental coverage. The name of the game is for the carrier to pay for the least expensive service option, regardless of which one best serves the patient's needs.

For example, let us say that you need to have one of your upper front teeth replaced. A removable partial denture will cost $500 while a fixed bridge will cost $1,400. Most current insurance carriers pay about 50 percent of the cost of dental services based on their usual and customary rate (UCR) for your geographic area. You pay the other 50 percent (also called a copayment). That means that, in this case, the insurance carrier would be obligated to pay either 50 percent of $500 ($250) or 50 percent of $1,400 ($700). These figures assume that the fees charged were the UCR for your area. If they participate in the "new approach," they will pay $250 for the removable partial instead of $700 for the bridge. It would then be your responsibility to pay the difference of $450 if you wanted the fixed bridge, the preferable choice from the dental provider's standpoint. Before you start any basic or major treatment it is always best to have your dentist send a predetermination plan to your insurance company so you will know ahead exactly what will be covered. It is important to remember that predeterminations from insurance companies are not a guarantee of payment. All insurance companies reserve the right to deny payment of claims that their dental consultant has reviewed, if the completed treatment does not satisfy their guidelines. *It is very important for patients to remember all treatment decisions should be made by you and your dentist, not you and your insurance company.* Dental benefit coverage should be taken into account, but should not be the deciding factor in your choice of treatment. It is common for plans to exclude or discourage necessary dental procedures (e.g., sealants, adult orthodontics, and specialty referrals). Some plans are designed to allow coverage only for the least expensive way to treat a dental need. This is certainly not in the best interest of your long-term oral health care.

Patients should know that it is illegal to ask a dentist to send a claim for reimbursement to an insurance company if treatment is started before the coverage begins or if the treatment has not yet been completed. In other words, your dentist cannot send in your claim for payment on a crown until the crown has been placed in your mouth. If you decide not to get the crown after the dentist has already had the crown made, he can only charge a fee for his time spent and lab costs. He cannot send in charges using the code to identify placement of a crown.

The ADA has a list of universal insurance codes that dentists use when sending in a claim. All insurance companies accept these codes to identify procedures when processing claims. It is important for patients to realize that their insurance policy is a contract between them and their insurance carrier. The insurance carrier is responsible to you, not the dentist. Likewise, patients, not their insurance carriers, are responsible for any fees the dentist charges for treatment. If the insurance carrier does not pay for the treatment, the patient is still responsible for the charges. Of course, dentists in managed care plans must abide by any contractual agreements they have made with an insurance company. Dentists who offer to carry the amount covered by a patient's insurance carrier and file the insurance claim for the patient are doing this as a courtesy. Many dentists today, due to the high overhead involved with handling insurance claims, request their patients pay in full at each visit and give them a form to attach to their insurance claim so they can handle their own insurance. On the average, claims take between 30 and 90 days to be processed. Check with your dentist to determine his policy regarding this matter.

If both you and your spouse have dental coverage you can coordinate your benefits. After the primary carrier has paid benefits for a procedure the *explanation of benefits* (EOB) is sent to the secondary carrier. Both plans must cover the enrollee, the spouse, and dependents in the family before coordination of benefits can occur. It is important to note that when benefits are coordinated from both plans the coverage will never exceed 100 percent. When determining who is the primary carrier for your children, most plans consider the spouse who has a birthday occurring earlier in the calendar year as primary. However, this determination depends on the regulations in your state so it is necessary to get this clarified from your insurance company.

Patients sometimes do not understand why dentists are reluctant to join managed care plans. According to Ms. Marge Feldman in the August 1, 1995, *ADA News*, capitation plans have failed because recent surveys show that general dentists have an overhead of about 67 percent compared to an overhead of only 25 to 30 percent in medicine. Most capitation plans ask the general dentist to discount their fees 10 to 30 percent. Recent surveys indicate the cost of implementing ADA and CDC infection control guidelines and the compliance with Occupational Safety and Health Administration guidelines has resulted in a cost of $9.31 per patient to the dentist. That is more than many capitation plans pay a general dentist per month in premiums for treating patients in these plans. Remember, only part of the premium you pay each month on a managed care plan goes to the dentist. The balance of the money is kept by the carrier for administrative costs. The carrier also has to have some portion of the premium for profit.

Insurance companies have great success selling their capitation dental programs because they are able to offer subscribers less costly dental programs that include the same services as more costly plans. Basically, the insurance companies use the general dentists to help sell their capitation programs to employers. Dentists today have such a high overhead to operate their offices that very few can afford to cut their fees 10 to 30 percent without compromising on the quality of care they deliver to their patients. I feel Dr. Michael McMunn expressed the situation quite well when he wrote in the April–June 1985 *Virginia Dental Journal*: "It is one thing when a patient says, 'I can't afford it,' but another when the dentist says, 'I can't afford to do it.'" There is potential for these plans to encourage substandard dental care through under utilization if they are not handled properly.

Dental insurance coverage for individuals is not readily available because dental needs are very predictable. Insurance companies know that you are not going to want to pay more for the premiums than the actual treatment will cost. Therefore, they stand to lose money on each policy they write because you are likely to discontinue the plan after all the major treatment is completed because the premiums are more expensive than the benefits. Dental policies available for individuals usually involve a monthly fee paid to the insurance company for access to a list of dentists who will agree to reduce their fee schedule to members of the plan. Payment for treatment is paid directly to the dentist. The dentist benefits by getting the referrals, but he does not receive any payment from the insurance company. The insurance company gets the premium for matching the individual with the dentist.

Before you choose a plan always find out what provisions have been made if you need emergency treatment. If you are on a managed care plan it is necessary to know where to call if you cannot reach your assigned dentist. Ask your dental insurance company what benefits are considered "emergency treatment" and what level of reimbursement you can expect for these procedures. Some health insurance plans have limited dental coverage. Usually the coverage only includes certain surgical procedures and accidents. It is important to have your insurance company clarify the extent of your coverage if you have this benefit included in your health insurance plan. These benefits are not designed to take the place of dental health insurance. Dental plans usually exclude treatment that is already covered under a companies medical plan. Sometimes plans also have *exclusions* (procedures not covered on the plan) that include necessary dental treatment (e.g. sealants, adult ortho-dontics, specialist referrals, and preexisting conditions). It is not uncom-mon for plans to exclude treatment by family members. Patients need to be aware of the exclusions and limitations on their plan, but they should not let them determine their treatment decisions. Remember, the level of coverage included in a dental plan determines the premium charged to the enrollee. Therefore, the inexpensive plans provide only for the least expensive way to treat a dental need, regardless of the best treatment your dentist recommends.

As you can see there are many options when it comes to dental insurance. If you have questions about your particular plan it is best to contact either your insurance broker, if you are self-employed, or the insurance representative at your job. Take your time and make sure you understand the plan *before* you make a commitment.

16

What Can You Expect to Pay for Dental Services?

I n October 1985, *Dental Economics* magazine reported that the Federal Trade Commission's Bureau of Competition would henceforth allow the American Dental Association (ADA) to conduct fee surveys in the United States. In the past the ADA had done annual studies of dental fees charged by dentists in the United States, but the FTC would not allow this information to be distributed or published. It was the Bureau's position that the ADA's data could be used to aid dentists in fixing fees and would thus be in violation of antitrust laws. In the new ruling, the FTC stated that it would now permit fee surveys to be conducted so that patients and dentists could evaluate the dental fees charged. In order to insure that the surveys did not violate antitrust laws, the FTC required them to be voluntary, and the results had to include a fee range rather than a set price.

Since the 1985 ruling, the ADA and several dental-related trade magazines in the United States have begun to publish the results of fee surveys they conduct annually. Most of the current data included in the tables related to this chapter on fees for the United States has been taken from the dental fees survey published in the September–October 1996 *Dental Practice and Finance* magazine, Medec Dental Communications, Northfield, Illinois. This data is a good representation of the currently available information in dental fee surveys for the United States.

In this particular survey, 3,500 dentists nationwide were sent the survey forms, and the response rate was 36.8 percent (considered very good). For purposes of analyzing the data, the United States was divided into nine regions. All regions were well represented in the returned surveys. More than three out of four of the returned surveys (83.7 percent) came from general practitioners, and nearly all of them (96.8 percent) stated they were in private practice. Nine out of ten respondents (89 percent) stated they were practicing full time (defined as 32 or more hours per week), and three out of four (76.5 percent) declared themselves as sole proprietors.

It is important to note dental fees for an area are directly impacted by the cost of living in that region. The overhead expenses (rent, salaries, utilities, laboratory costs, and supplies) are very high for the dentists in the areas with the highest fees. Not unlike surveys in the past, this survey has again consistently demonstrated that fees in the New England and Pacific regions of the United States are the highest. The fees in the central regions, particularly the East South Central area, seem to be the lowest. Likewise, dentists in the suburbs of large metropolitan areas (500,000+) consistently charge the highest fees, and providers in the towns with populations under 20,000 consistently charge the least. This makes sense because the cost of living (overhead) is much higher in the suburbs around large metropolitan areas than in small towns.

All three of the tables provided for the United States consist of the same set of frequently performed dental procedures. To further aid in clarity, a brief description of each procedure and its ADA universal insurance code is furnished in tables 1 and 3. (The universal insurance codes enable dentists to have a standardized language to describe specific dental procedures.) All of the figures used in these tables are based on the median fee (national average) for each procedure. According to Mr. Bob Kehoe in the September–October 1995 *Dental Practice and Finance* article on dental fees, a median fee is "the exact middle of all responses nationally; this means that half the respondents charged more than this amount and half charged less." Therefore, when you look at the fees in your area for each procedure remember that half the dentists in your area charge more than this fee and half charge less. It is unlikely your dentist will charge exactly the fee listed for any included procedure. These fees are just meant to be used as a guide for each region, not the exact fee your dentist charges. Many factors, such as cost of living in your area and the size of the city where you live, impact the dental fees. Also, you must remember that fees charged to patients who are in managed care plans are usually 20 to 40 percent lower than the fees being quoted by dentists in the area to patients who are not in managed care programs.

All of the tables included in the appendix are comparisons of fees for the same specific procedures. The tables contain a group of some of the most commonly performed procedures performed in dental offices.

Table 1 compares the median fees (national average) in the United States for selected procedures in 1985, 1995, and 1996. It is interesting to note that the increase in dental fees is very close to the increase in the cost of other consumer goods and services. This has been true for over a decade and, presumably, will continue to be true.

Table 2 compares the median fees (national average) in the United States for selected procedures in 1996 with those of 1985. The United States is divided into nine regions for purposes of comparison. The states included in each region are as follows (see figure 8):

New England (Connecticut, Maine, Massachusetts, New Hampshire, Rhode Island, and Vermont)

Middle Atlantic (New Jersey, New York, and Pennsylvania)

East North Central (Illinois, Indiana, Ohio, Michigan, and Wisconsin)

West North Central (Iowa, Kansas, Minnesota, Missouri, Nebraska, North Dakota, and South Dakota)

South Atlantic (Delaware, Florida, Georgia, Maryland, North Carolina, South Carolina, Virginia, Washington D.C., and West Virginia)

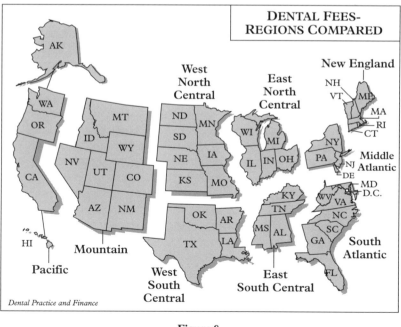

Figure 8

East South Central (Alabama, Kentucky, Mississippi, and Tennessee)

West South Central (Arkansas, Louisiana, Oklahoma, and Texas)

Mountain (Arizona, Colorado, Idaho, Montana, Nevada, New Mexico, Utah, and Wyoming)

Pacific (Alaska, California, Hawaii, Oregon, and Washington)

Table 3 compares dental fees in the United States for 1996 by quartile rankings. The national average median fees are located in the first column. Essentially, the dental fees included in the bottom quartile (25 percent) column are the small towns with populations less than 20,000 and the areas in the central regions of the United States. The fees included in the top quartile (25 percent) column are the suburbs of the large metropolitan areas (500,000+) and the Pacific and New England areas of the United States. As we have already mentioned, the dentists in the higher cost of living areas have a higher overhead and the fees are higher. The dentists in smaller areas have the lower fees because the cost of living (overhead) is less.

Before you decide to rush to the smaller towns to get dental treatment do not lose sight of the fact that the larger metropolitan areas offer a far greater range of dentists and dental specialists than the smaller towns. The cost of services might be less in the smaller towns, but the choices and expertise available cannot be addressed by the statistical data in the tables.

These tables do not include Canadian fees. Appendix C includes names of and contact information for Canadian dental associations.

TABLE 1
COMPARISON OF NATIONAL MEDIAN[1] FEES FOR
DENTAL SERVICES (1985[2], 1995[3], 1996[4]) IN THE
UNITED STATES

Procedure with ADA Code	1985[2]	1995[3]	1996[4]
Initial oral exam (00110)	$17	$26	$30[5]
Periodic oral exam (00120)	$12	$20	$20
Panoramic film (00330)	$31	$50	$51
Full-mouth X rays (00210)	$36	$63[5]	$60
Bitewing X rays (00274)	$13	$26	$27
Prophylaxis (Perio scaling with gingival irritation, adult) (01110)	$25	$42	$44
Prophylaxis (child) (01120)	$19	$30	$31
Sealant (per tooth) (01351)	$12[5]	$22	$24
Fluoride treatment (excluding prophylaxis) (01203)	$12	$20[5]	$20[5]
Amalgam restoration (one surface), permanent tooth (02140)	$26	$56[5]	$56[5]
Amalgam restoration (two surfaces), permanent tooth (02150)	$37	$65	$66
Amalgam restoration (three surfaces), permanent tooth (02160)	$46	$77	$80
Composite resin restoration (anterior) one surface, permanent tooth (02330)	$32	$60	$65
Composite resin restoration (anterior) two surfaces, permanent tooth (02331)	$44	$78	$80
Composite resin restoration (posterior) two surfaces, permanent tooth (02385)	[6]	$85	$90
Full gold crown (02790)	$343	$550[5]	$550[5]
Porcelain fused to high noble metal crown (02750)	$338	$545	$550
Porcelain/ceramic crown (02740)	$332[5]	$535	$550
Stainless steel crown (prefabricated) (02931)	$80	$146[5]	$146[5]
Post and core (prefabricated), in addition to crown (02954)	$93	$140	$140
Post and core (cast), in addition to crown (02952)	$116[5]	$175	$175
Recement crown (02920)	$21	$45[5]	$45[5]
Labial veneer, laminate (chairside) (02960)	$90	$175	$191
Labial veneer, porcelain laminate, lab (02962)	$195[5]	$400	$429
Extraction (simple), single tooth (07110)	$32	$62	$65
Root canal therapy, one canal (anterior), excluding final restoration (03310)	$166	$295	$300
Root canal therapy, 2 canals (biscuspid), excluding final restoration (03320)	$210	$352	$375

TABLE 1 (cont.)

Procedure with ADA Code	1985[2]	1995[3]	1996[4]
Root canal therapy, 3 canals (molar), excluding final restoration (03330)	$273	$450	$475
Bleaching of endodontically treated tooth (03960)	$47[5]	$100	$100
Periodontal scaling/root planing, quadrant (04341)	$54	$105	$113
Implant maintenance (06080)	[6]	$90	$80
Complete upper denture (05110)	$461	$684	$700
Complete lower denture (05120)	$461	$682	$700
Upper denture reline—chairside (05730)	$55[5]	$144	$150
Bleaching—per arch (chairside) (09999)	$80[5]	$175	$175
Fabrication of athletic mouth guards (09941)	$35[5]	$75	$85
Occlusal guards, by report (09940)	[6]	$204	$225

[1] The median fee is the exact middle of all responses nationally; this means that half the respondents charged more than this amount and half charged less.

[2] Reprinted with permission, Copyright 1985, *Dental Management*, Harcourt Brace Jovanovich Healthcare Publications.

[3] Reprinted with permission, Copyright 1995, *Dental Practice and Finance*, Medec Dental Communications, Northfield, Ill.

[4] Reprinted with permission, Copyright 1996, *Dental Practice and Finance*, Medec Dental Communications, Northfield, Ill.

[5] Data was obtained from a combination of sources

[6] Data not available

TABLE 2
1996[1] (1985[2]) NATIONAL MEDIAN[3] REGIONAL COST ANALYSIS FOR DENTAL SERVICES IN THE UNITED STATES

Procedure	New England	Middle Atlantic	East North Central	West North Central	South Atlantic
Initial oral exam	$35[4] (19)	$32[4] (19)	$28[4] (14)	$23[4] (12)	$28[4] (17)
Periodic oral exam	$22 (13)	$23 (13)	$20 (10)	$18 (10)	$23 (11)
Panoramic film	$65 (38)	$55 (33)	$52 (33)	$48 (29)	$51 (27)
Full-mouth X rays	$65[4] (39)	$65[4] (37)	$59[4] (35)	$55[4] (34)	$60[4] (33)
Bitewing X rays	$30 (14)	$29 (13)	$25 (12)	$24 (12)	$25 (12)
Prophylaxis (adult)	$49 (27)	$49 (26)	$40 (23)	$36 (21)	$40 (23)
Prophylaxis (child)	$35 (20)	$34 (18)	$28 (17)	$25 (14)	$30 (17)
Sealant (per tooth)	$25 (15[4])	$25 (16[4])	$21 (13[4])	$19 (10[4])	$24 (13[4])
Fluoride treatment	$21[4] (14)	$21[4] (13)	$18[4] (12)	$15[4] (10)	$17[4] (10)
1-surface amalgam	$59[4] (26)	$55[4] (24)	$49[4] (24)	$474 (23)	$51[4] (25)

TABLE 2 (cont.)

Procedure	New England	Middle Atlantic	East North Central	West North Central	South Atlantic
2-surface amalgam	$70 (38)	$68 (36)	$60 (33)	$57 (34)	$68 (34)
3-surface amalgam	$85 (48)	$85 (48)	$75 (42)	$69 (42)	$82 (43)
1-surface composite resin, anterior	$70 (30)	$65 (30)	$59 (29)	$54 (28)	$65 (29)
2-surface composite resin, anterior	$85 (43)	$85 (45)	$75 (39)	$68 (38)	$82 (39)
2-surface composite resin, posterior	$91 $(^5)$	$90 $(^5)$	$85 $(^5)$	$82 $(^5)$	$85 $(^5)$
Full gold crown	$656^4 (404)	$616^4 (378)	$5184 (326)	$469^4 (288)	$549^4 (336)
Porcelain fused to metal crown	$648 (395)	$588 (379)	$500 (321)	$460 (283)	$540 (322)
Porcelain/ceramic crown	$650 ($389^4$)	$600 ($373^4$)	$512 ($315^4$)	$487 ($277^4$)	$550 ($316^4$)
Stainless steel crown (prefabricated)	$174^4 (93)	$165^4 (96)	$139^4 (76)	$144^4 (62)	$140^4 (79)
Post and core (prefabricated)	$165 (112)	$150 (106)	$135 (94)	$120 (76)	$135 (84)
Post and core (cast)	$200 ($135^4$)	$186 ($129^4$)	$175 ($117^4$)	$150 ($99^4$)	$157 ($110^4$)
Recement crown	$53^4 (25)	$44^4 (22)	$43^4 (20)	$40^4 (18)	$41^4 (20)
Labial veneer, laminate (chairside)	$175 (84)	$200 (101)	$162 (80)	$165 (78)	$183 (90)
Labial veneer (lab) porcelain laminate	$450 ($189^4$)	$400 ($206^4$)	$400 ($185^4$)	$375 ($183^4$)	$450 ($195^4$)
Extraction, single tooth	$75 (35)	$75 (33)	$61 (28)	$54 (28)	$65 (28)
Root canal therapy, one canal	$348 (181)	$325 (181)	$289 (157)	$255 (138)	$310 (161)
Root canal therapy, two canals	$428 (244)	$398 (233)	$350 (199)	$308 (170)	$385 (204)
Root canal therapy, three canals	$560 (340)	$500 (311)	$450 (257)	$393 (313)	$475 (265)
Bleaching of an endo-dontically treated tooth	$100 $(^5)$	$100 $(^5)$	$87 $(^5)$	$80 $(^5)$	$95 $(^5)$
Periodontal scaling/ root planing (quadrant)	$125 (58)	$122 (61)	$125 (53)	$109 (44)	$120 (54)
Implant maintenance	$100 $(^5)$	$117 $(^5)$	$65 $(^5)$	$53 $(^5)$	$75 $(^5)$
Dentures:					
Complete upper	$757 (476)	$750 (449)	$650 (444)	$640 (447)	$675 (418)
Complete lower	$757 (476)	$750 (449)	$650 (444)	$629 (447)	$698 (418)

TABLE 2 (cont.)

Procedure	New England	Middle Atlantic	East North Central	West North Central	South Atlantic
Reline—upper denture (chairside)	$162 ([5])	$150 ([5])	$150 ([5])	$125 ([5])	$140 ([5])
Bleaching—per arch (chairside)	$190 ([5])	$200 ([5])	$170 ([5])	$150 ([5])	$175 ([5])
Fabrication of athletic mouth guard	$78 ([5])	$125 ([5])	$72 ([5])	$45 ([5])	$89 ([5])
Occlusal guards, by report	$225 ([5])	$225 ([5])	$225 ([5])	$175 ([5])	$250 ([5])

TABLE 2 (cont.)

Procedure	East South Central	West South Central	Mountain	Pacific
Initial oral exam	$23[4] (14)	$25[4] (16)	$27[4] (16)	$37[4] (19)
Periodic oral exam	$17 (10)	$20 (12)	$21 (11)	$29 (15)
Panoramic film	$49 (32)	$45 (30)	$49 (29)	$60 (34)
Full-mouth X rays	$55 (34)	$55 (33)	$60 (33)	$75 (42)
Bitewing X rays	$24 (12)	$25 (13)	$27 (12)	$38 (19)
Perio scaling (adult)	$36 (22)	$40 (26)	$45 (26)	$58 (32)
Prophylaxis (child)	$27 (17)	$30 (19)	$32 (18)	$45 (26)
Sealant (per tooth)	$20 (8[4])	$22 (11[4])	$22 (12[4])	$30 (17[4])
Fluoride treatment	$14[4] (10)	$14[4] (11)	$17[4] (9)	$26[4] (15)
1-surface amalgam	$46[4] (25)	$54[4] (29)	$55[4] (27)	$70[4] (34)
2-surface amalgam	$55 (33)	$65 (40)	$69 (38)	$87 (44)
3-surface amalgam	$67 (41)	$79 (51)	$82 (49)	$100 (54)
1-surface composite resin, anterior	$52 (29)	$63 (35)	$65 (32)	$90 (43)
2-surface composite resin, anterior	$65 (40)	$80 (45)	$80 (44)	$120 (60)
2-surface composite resin, posterior	$71 ([5])	$90 ([5])	$85 ([5])	$125 ([5])
Full gold crown	$449[4] (299)	$503[4] (345)	$511[4] (313)	$601[4] (362)
Porcelain fused to metal crown	$454 (284)	$495 (343)	$525 (320)	$600 (359)
Porcelain/ceramic crown	$456 (278[4])	$518 (337[4])	$548 (314[4])	$600 (353[4])
Stainless steel crown (prefabricated)	$115[4] (77)	$129[4] (69)	$129[4] (86)	$156[4] (83)
Post and core (prefabricated)	$120 (83)	$129 (90)	$125 (78)	$150 (93)

REGIONAL FEES
1996[1], (1985)[2]

Procedure	East South Central	West South Central	Mountain	Pacific
Post and core (cast)	$131 (106[4])	$155 (113[4])	$160 (101[4])	$200 (116[4])
Recement crown	$36[4] (17)	$38[4] (21)	$45[4] (19)	$56[4] (27)
Labial veneer, laminate (chairside)	$162 (77)	$199 (95)	$152 (98)	$250 (100)
Labial veneer (lab) porcelain laminate	$355 (182[4])	$420 (200[4])	$445 (203[4])	$525 (205[4])
Extraction (single tooth)	$50 (27)	$60 (33)	$63 (32)	$85 (38)
Root canal therapy, one canal	$265 (151)	$281 (162)	$300 (157)	$370 (186)
Root canal therapy, two canals	$325 (189)	$335 (202)	$368 (197)	$440 (233)
Root canal therapy, three canals	$400 (242)	$425 (258)	$453 (252)	$545 (298)
Bleaching of an endodontically treated tooth	$95 ([5])	$91 ([5])	$100 ([5])	$120 ([5])
Periodontal scaling/root planing (per quadrant)	$94 (54)	$100 (55)	$114 (49)	$130 (53)
Implant maintenance	$65([5])	$65([5])	$86([5])	$112([5])
Dentures:				
Complete upper	$562 (409)	$670 (527)	$675 (485)	$800 (507)
Complete lower	$562 (409)	$656 (527)	$675 (485)	$800 (507)
Reline—upper denture (chairside)	$110 ([5])	$142 ([5])	$110 ([5])	$172 ([5])
Bleaching—per arch (chairside)	$150 ([5])	$180 ([5])	$150 ([5])	$175 ([5])
Fabrication of athletic mouth guard	$80 ([5])	$80 ([5])	$93 ([5])	$140 ([5])
Occlusal guards, by report	$175 ([5])	$225 ([5])	$230 ([5])	$275 ([5])

[1] Reprinted with permission, Copyright 1996, *Dental Practice and Finance*, Medec Dental Communications, Northfield, Ill.

[2] Reprinted with permission, Copyright 1985, *Dental Management*, Harcourt Brace Jovanovich Healthcare Publications.

[3] The median fee is the exact middle of all responses nationally; this means that half the respondents charged more than this amount and half charged less.

[4] Data obtained from a combination of sources

[5] Data not available

TABLE 3
1996[1] NATIONAL FEE SURVEY:
QUARTILE RANKINGS FOR THE UNITED STATES

Procedure with ADA Code	National Average (Median[2] Fee)	Bottom Quartile	Top Quartile
Initial oral exam (00110)	$30	[4]	[4]
Periodic oral exam (00120)	$20	$15	$35
Panoramic film (00330)	$51	$41	$70
Full mouth X rays (00210)	$60	$45	$80
Bitewing X rays (00274)	$27	$20	$40
Prophylaxis (adult) (01110)	$44	$34	$60
Prophylaxis (child) (01120)	$31	$23	$48
Sealant (per tooth) (01351)	$24	$16	$32
Fluoride treatment (excluding prophylaxis) (01203)	$20[3]	[4]	[4]
Amalgam restoration (permanent tooth), one surface (02140)	$56[3]	[4]	[4]
Amalgam restoration (permanent tooth) two surfaces (02150)	$66	$50	$90
Amalgam restoration (permanent tooth) three surfaces (02160)	$80	$63	$106
Composite resin restoration (permanent) one surface, anterior (02330)	$65	$48	$90
Composite resin restoration (permanent) two surfaces, anterior (02331)	$80	$60	$120
Composite resin restoration (permanent) two surfaces, posterior (02385)	$90	$65	$139
Full gold crown (02790)	$550[3]	[4]	[4]
Porcelain fused to high noble metal crown (02750)	$550	$450	$675
Porcelain/ceramic crown (02740)	$550	$450	$675
Stainless steel crown (prefabricated) (02954)	$146[3]	[4]	[4]
Post and core (prefabricated), in addition to crown (02954)	$140	$95	$195
Post and core (cast), in addition to crown (02950)	$175	$117	$250

TABLE 3 (cont.)

Procedure with ADA Code	National Average (Median[2] Fee)	Bottom Quartile	Top Quartile
Recement crown (02920)	$45[3]	[4]	[4]
Labial veneer, laminate (chairside) (02960)	$191	$109	$350
Labial veneer, porcelain laminate (lab) (02962)	$429	$300	$593
Extraction, simple (single tooth) (07110)	$65	$48	$91
Root canal therapy, one canal (anterior), excluding final restoration (03310)	$300	$226	$400
Root canal therapy, 2 canals (bicuspid), excluding final restoration (03320)	$375	$286	$485
Root canal therapy, 3 canals (molar), excluding final restoration (03330)	$475	$375	$600
Bleaching of endodontically treated tooth (03960)	$100	$50	$175
Periodontal scaling/root planing (quadrant) (04341)	$113	$75	$150
Implant maintenance (06080)	$80	$45	$165
Dentures: Complete upper denture (05110)	$700	$515	$950
Complete lower denture (05120)	$700	$515	$950
Reline upper denture (chairside) (05730)	$150	$85	$215
Bleaching—per arch (chairside) (09999)	$175	$100	$275
Fabrication of athletic mouth guards (09941)	$85	$30	$180
Occlusal guards, by report (09940)	$225	$90	$400

[1] Reprinted with permission, Copyright 1996, *Dental Practice and Finance*, Medec Dental Communications, Northfield, Ill.

[2] The median fee is the exact middle of all responses nationally; this means that half the respondents charged more than this amount and half charged less.

[3] Data was obtained from a combination of sources

[4] Data not available

Conclusion

The information covered in this book includes most of the usual dental procedures and terminology that you might encounter in discussing your dental treatment with your dentist. A panel of general dentists and specialists, each with 10 to 30 years clinical experience, has carefully checked all the information in this book to insure that the latest techniques being used in private practice at this writing have been included.

No longer do you, as a dental consumer, need to go to the dentist and not know what he is talking about or what questions you should ask. The specific techniques your dentist uses might vary slightly; however, the general principles will be basically the same as described in this book.

The authors wrote this book with the intent that the reader would use it as a reference text. It is not intended to be a book that is read once, digested, and all the details remembered. The book is written in simple, readable terminology. In addition, specific areas of interest about which the reader is interested can be readily found in designated chapters (e.g. orthodontics).

If your dentist says you need a silver filling, the book index can help you find the pages where silver fillings are discussed. The glossary defines terms in the book that you need to have clarified or do not know. And the topics that need debunking are discussed (e.g. mercury toxicity) in the issues section.

This book also contains fee tables with average fee charges for specific services in different parts of the United States. These fee tables should be used with the knowledge that they only represent averages. This means that some dentists may charge more while an equal number charge less.

We are in a new era, even for dentists, in terms of the innovative delivery systems that have emerged (HMOs, CPOs, etc.). Only time will determine if these systems are good or bad for the dental consumer. Insurance companies have gotten into the picture and are increasing their influence. This book should help you to choose a good policy for yourself and your family.

Dentists today spend about four years in dental school. No consumer can learn in one book what it took their dentist four years to understand. However, this book can help you comprehend what your dentist is proposing for your dental treatment. The dentist-patient relationship is one of trust.

On any given day some new dental device or procedure is discovered. Dentistry changes but no dentist has a corner on the market of expertise or the use of new techniques. If you come across a "new" idea, ask how long it has been used, and whether it is recognized by the American Dental Association.

Basic Terms and Definitions

abscess An infection in the jawbone from either dead pulp in the tooth or a periodontal pocket around the tooth.

abutment A support (anchor) tooth on either side of the space where a tooth is missing.

acid etch A technique whereby a tooth is first treated with a mild acid solution, and then washed and dried. This makes the tooth surface rough (etched), thus allowing some tooth-colored materials to adhere to the tooth surface.

acquired immune deficiency syndrome (AIDS) This disease is caused by the retrovirus known as HIV type 1. The modes of transmission are sexual (vaginal fluids, semen), blood or blood products, and perinatal transmission from an infected mother to the fetus or to the newborn at birth. Infection results in progressive immune dysregulation, dysfunction, and deficiency.

Actisite A tetracycline-impregnated fiber used in treating periodontal pockets.

ADA An acronym for the American Dental Association.

AIDS The acronym for "acquired immune deficiency syndrome." The early symptoms of this disease manifest in the mouth, so they can often be detected by your dentist.

alloy A combination of precious and semiprecious materials (e.g. mercury, silver, copper, tin, zinc, gold, chromium, and nickel) used in tooth restorations (e.g. crowns, inlays, and onlays).

alveolar bone The bone that supports the teeth in the jaw.

231
▲

amalgam   A silver filling material that contains alloys of mercury, silver, copper, tin, and sometimes zinc. It is still the most common type of dental restoration.

amalgam bonding   A new type of amalgam recently developed. Instead of placing the amalgam directly into the prepared tooth, a layer of resin is put in first. The resin bonds to the tooth, and the amalgam bonds to the resin. This makes the restoration stronger, and helps eliminate tooth sensitivity.

American Dental Association (ADA)   The national organization for organized dentistry in the United States. The national ADA headquarters in Chicago is responsible for advising state and local dental societies about policies of state and national interest.

American Dental Association Seal of Acceptance   The only labeling on dental products that assures the consumer of their safety and efficacy, and that the manufacturer's claims are accurate.

analgesic   A medication that produces an absence of the sensation of pain. Aspirin and Tylenol are common analgesics that provide relief from pain.

anesthesia   The loss of all sensation in an area through the action of drugs. Anesthesia produces a numbing effect. Common local anesthetics are Xylocaine and Carbocaine.

anterior   Pertaining to the front, as in anterior teeth.

antibiotic   A medication given to aid the body's defenses in fighting infectious diseases. Examples include penicillin, erythromycin, etc.

antifluoridationist   People opposed to the addition of fluoride to public drinking water.

apex   The tip end of the tooth root. The part of the root farthest from the crown or chewing surface of the tooth.

aphthous ulcers   *See* recurrent aphthous ulcers.

apical curettage   The surgical removal of infection in the bone around the root apex with a small spoon-shaped surgical instrument.

apical foramen   The exit point of the pulp tissue from the lower end of the root.

apicoectomy   Surgical removal of the root apex, including the removal of any surrounding diseased bone.

appliance   A broad dental term meaning any dental device that serves a useful purpose. Such devices include dentures, orthodontic bands, etc.

arbitration committee   A peer review.

arch   A dental ridge; referring to the bony elevation from which the teeth erupt in the upper or lower jaw.

arch wire   An orthodontic wire used as an aid in straightening teeth.

articulator A device used by a dentist or dental laboratory technician to simulate the natural action of the jaws when biting. Its function is to aid in the fabrication of dental appliances.

attachment A device or tissue that fastens to another device, tooth, etc. (e.g. a clasp on a partial denture that enables the partial to attach to an existing tooth).

atypical face pain (AFP) A condition most authorities feel may be caused by depression and anxiety. It is characterized by tenderness in the upper jaw at the root ends of the molars. Some authorities feel it may have a psychological origin.

audio-anesthesia A distraction technique to accomplish anesthesia. Listening to a radio or tape recorder, even watching television, has been used with some success.

avulsion A term used to describe a tooth that has been entirely knocked out of the socket.

"baby bottle" syndrome Decay in a child's teeth caused by frequent exposure to liquids containing sugars (e.g. milk, formula, fruit juice).

bacterial endocarditis A serious inflammation of the heart valves or tissues. The American Heart Association recommends a regime of antibiotics to be taken before any dental treatment to reduce the incidence of this problem.

band *See* orthodontic band.

base A material used in repairing deep cavities. In theory, bases thermally insulate and protect the pulp.

benign tumor A noninvasive (self-limiting) growth that is not malignant. It may or may not resolve itself.

Benzocaine A topical anesthetic used to create surface numbing of the dental injection site.

bicuspidization Making a molar into two bicuspids by surgically dividing the roots after root canal therapy.

biopsy Surgical removal of a tissue specimen to determine the types of cells present. This is often a screening for cancer.

bitewing An X-ray film that reveals the crowns of the teeth. This film is taken primarily to check for decay between teeth.

bleaching A technique that involves making the teeth lighter.

block anesthesia Anesthesia or numbness obtained by removing sensation from a major nerve trunk through a local anesthesic. Most commonly used in anesthetizing the lower jaw.

board-certified specialist A specialist who is a diplomate of the American board for his dental specialty.

board-eligible specialist A dentist who has graduated from an advanced ADA-approved training program. A specialist who is not yet a diplomate of his specialty board.

bonding   A technique that involves removing a small amount of tooth structure and placing a thin covering over the top of the tooth to repair, protect, or return a discolored tooth to its natural color.

bone grafts   A method of regenerating lost bone by placing either human, synthetic, or freeze-dried (demineralized) bone in the area where the bone loss has occurred.

bony impaction   A condition whereby a tooth is not in proper position, and it cannot erupt.

bracket   *See* orthodontic bracket.

bridge   A tooth-replacing fixed appliance having one or more crowns that serve as an abutment to anchor the bridge to existing teeth when it is cemented into place.

bruxism   A "natural" grinding of the teeth to release tension. If the bruxism is severe and causes joint-related problems in the jaw, a general dentist or dental specialist should be consulted to aid in correcting the problem.

buccal   The surface of a tooth in contact with the cheek; opposite to the lingual surface.

burning mouth syndrome (BMS)   A condition characterized by a constant pain in both sides of the mouth, usually in multiple sites.

CAD/CAM (computer-aided design/computer-aided manufacture)   A system that enables the dentist to design and fabricate dental restorations at chairside in one appointment instead of using conventional methods for inlays, onlays, veneers, crowns, and bridges.

calcified   Hardened; this condition occurs when the soft tissue inside the tooth hardens from exposure to trauma or infection over a period of time.

calculus   This substance forms when plaque is allowed to remain on the teeth and harden.

canker sores   *See* recurrent aphthous ulcers.

cantilever bridge   A fixed bridge in which the pontic is the end member.

capitation   A method of reimbursement in dental benefit plans that requires the dentist to provide all necessary covered services to eligible members of the plan for a fixed per capita monthly payment, usually paid regardless of the services rendered. The dentist assumes the financial risk in these plans.

carcinoma   An oral cancer of the most serious type.

caries   The technical term used for tooth decay.

carrier   This is another term for the dental insurance company that offers dental insurance benefits to eligible members of the plan.

CDO   *See* contract dentist organization.

cementum   The thin, outermost mineralized layer covering the tooth root surface. The periodontal ligament attaches to this surface. When cementum is exposed, it can be very sensitive.

clasp   An "arm" of a partial denture. In most instances, it attaches to an abutment tooth to help in the stability and retention of a removable prosthetic device.

cleft lip   A birth defect that causes the lip to appear split; also called harelip.

cleft palate   A birth defect in which there is a direct opening between the roof of the mouth and the floor of the nose.

closed panel   A dental insurance plan that requires the patients to receive their dental care only from a dentist who has agreed to contractual terms dictated by the plan. These terms generally include providing treatment at reduced fees. Usually, only a limited number of dentists in an area are allowed to participate in a closed panel.

COBRA plan   Insurance coverage offered to an insured person at the time of termination of employment. The benefits are usually more limited and more expensive.

codeine   A pain-relieving prescription medicine (an analgesic). Codeine is frequently used in combination with Tylenol or aspirin.

Code of Ethics   The ADA's rule of conduct for dental professionals.

cold sores   *See* herpes simplex.

compliance   Following the instructions of your dentist. The degree of compliance by the patient directly relates to the success or failure of the treatment.

component dental society   A local dental society that is part of the national American Dental Association.

composite resin   A commonly used tooth-colored filling material made of glass, fillers, and resin used to restore teeth.

conscious sedation   Drug-induced relaxation in which a patient remains responsive to verbal commands. There is some question about the "fine line" between conscious sedation and unconscious sedation.

constituent dental society   A state dental society that is part of the national American Dental Association.

contact   The point at which two adjacent or opposing teeth meet or touch.

contract dentist organization (CDO)   A group of dentists under contract to provide services at a discounted rate in exchange for access to that population. Also known as a preferred provider organization (PPO).

conventional braces   Orthodontic appliances that have metal brackets on the outer surfaces of the teeth.

coordination of benefits   Utilizing the benefits of both spouses' dental plans for all members of the family when their coverage includes themselves each other, and dependent children in their family.

copayment   In dental insurance, that part of the fee for dental services that is not covered by dental insurance (i.e. the part the consumer must pay himself).

core material   The bulk material used in filling a root canal. The core material is usually gutta-percha, a soft, moldable, rubber base material. On rare occasions silver points are still used.

cracked tooth syndrome   Usually referring to a minute, long-standing vertical fracture (from crown to root tip) in a tooth.

crossbite   A type of malocclusion whereby the lower teeth extend to the outside of the upper teeth instead of being in proper alignment. This problem usually needs orthodontic intervention to correct.

crown   1. A "natural" crown is the uppermost portion of the tooth that projects above the gums. 2. A restoration for a badly decayed or fractured tooth that covers the entire remaining tooth to restore it to its original size and shape. It is fabricated from porcelain, porcelain fused to metal, or an alloy composed of a precious or a nonprecious metal.

crown lengthening   1. A surgical procedure that includes removing gum tissue to expose part of the root of the tooth so it can be used to support a full coverage restoration. 2. A procedure that involves attaching "space-age" wires made of super-elastic (nickel-titanium) material that causes the tooth to erupt by exerting steady, gentle pressure on the tooth. This is usually used on teeth that have broken off at the gum line.

cusp   One of the pointed projections that composes the chewing or biting surface of a tooth.

deciduous tooth   A "baby tooth" that will eventually be replaced by an adult tooth.

deductible   That initial payment each calendar year for dental services for which the patient is liable before the insurance company will pay any benefits.

defect   An area of bone loss in the jaw.

degenerative joint disease   A condition in the jaw joint caused by osteoarthritis or rheumatoid arthritis.

dental arch   The upper or lower dental ridge in the jawbone, with or without teeth.

dental assistant   The assistant to the dentist. A certified dental assistant (CDA) is an assistant who has passed an ADA certification exam. Usually, a CDA goes through an ADA-approved training program.

dental hygienist   A trained dental worker whose responsibility is to clean teeth, take X rays, and do preliminary oral exams. A registered dental hygienist (RDH) is a hygienist who has completed an ADA-approved training program and has passed an ADA certifying examination.

dental ridge   The bony, tissue-covered support for the teeth in either the upper or lower arch. When teeth are missing, the ridge becomes the support for the denture.

dental therapeutics   Any dental product that claims curative or preventive properties. These products are evaluated by the ADA for safety and effectiveness, and for accuracy of the claims of the manufacturer, before the ADA Seal is given to the product.

dentin   The mineralized tissue which comprises the bulk of the tooth. Dentin is found under the enamel of the crown and under the cementum of the root. Its structure is tubular.

dentinal tubules   The tiny tissue tubes that make up the dentin. These dentinal tubules have been called the "pathways to the pulp."

dentin bonding agent   A material that adheres to dentin and materials such as amalgam and composite resins to replace tooth structure and give added strength. An added benefit is that they seal the dentin tubules, preventing sensitivity.

dentin-etched fillings   A tooth-colored filling material for restoring teeth that is etched to the dentin of the tooth with a mild acid.

denture   A removable plasticlike prosthetic appliance that replaces either all or part of a patient's missing teeth.

denture adhesive   Products sold over the counter to help make dentures fit more tightly on the dental ridge; essentially a soft temporary relining of the inside of the denture base.

denturism   The practice of and services offered by legally recognized lab technicians known as "denturists."

denturist   A laboratory technician legally able to make, fit, and adjust dentures for patients without the supervision or guidance of a trained dentist.

dependent   The spouse or child of a subsriber to a dental health plan who is eligible for dental benefits.

digital imaging radiovisiography (RVG)   A direct replacement for X-ray film with a sensor (an electronic image receptor) linked to a computer. Instead of capturing the image on an emulsion, an electronic chip called a CCD (charged coupled device) is used. This technique enables X rays to be taken with about 10 percent of the exposure to radiation needed for traditional X rays that capture images on an emulsion.

diplomate A certified dental specialist who has passed all phases of his specialty certifying board exams. This is the highest level of specialty attainment in dentistry.

direct pulp capping The procedure in which a material, usually calcium hydroxide or one of its compounds, is placed directly on a pulpal exposure to protect the sensitive pulp.

direct reimbursement plan An arrangement whereby an employer pays for dental fees incurred by his employee(s). The levels of coverage are based on the amount of dental expenditure in a plan year instead of categories of treatment.

disclosing solution A red chemical solution that reveals areas that you missed in your usual brushing.

distal The surface of a tooth farthest from the midline; opposite the mesial.

DMF index An index used to measure your dental health. This is a record of teeth that are decayed, missing, or filled.

double abutment The use of two adjacent teeth instead of a single tooth as support for fixed bridges or partial dentures.

dry socket An extraction site that fails to heal properly. It usually causes discomfort to the patient.

electronic dental anesthesia (EDA) A noninvasive technique that uses a targeted pain blocking signal to penetrate the tissue at the treatment site.

enamel The most highly mineralized tissue in the body. The natural tooth crown is composed of enamel. Below the enamel is dentin.

endodontic implants A technique utilizing an existing tooth by placing a metal post down the root canal of the tooth and extending into the bone.

endodontic retreatment Removal of previously placed root canal filling material that is failing and replacement of it with a new root filling material.

endodontics The dental specialty concerned with the diagnosis, prevention, treatment and causes of diseases of the dental pulp and the tissues at the root apex.

endodontic therapy A term used synonymously for root canal therapy.

endosteal A type of implant that is placed directly into the jawbone.

epinephrine A vasoconstrictor used with many anesthetic solutions. It restricts bleeding during surgery and maintains the anesthetic in the operative site. It should be used with caution in patients with heart disease.

erythroplakia A precancerous reddish-colored lesion found in the mouth.

exclusions Procedures not covered under the plan.

exclusive provider organization (EPO) Subscribers and dependents who belong to this type of dental benefits program do not receive any benefits if they are not treated by dentists who are members of the EPO.

explanation of benefits (EOB) A form generated by an insurance company that is sent to the enrollee and the providing dentist that explains both payment of benefits and denials of coverage.

extraction The removal of all or part of a tooth.

facial The surface of a tooth that lies against the inside of the cheek. This term is usually used for the front surfaces of anterior (front) teeth.

Federal Trade Commission A federal agency that regulates business practices, including those of the dental profession.

fee for service A method of reimbursement in dental benefit plans whereby benefits are paid to the patient or the dentist according to the services provided. The fees paid for the services are determined by usual and customary (UC) limitations, a table of allowances, fee schedules, or on the basis of the dentist's usual full fee. No financial risk is assumed by the dentist in these plans.

fever blisters *See* herpes simplex.

file A fine, tapered instrument used by a dentist to clean out pulpal tissue remnants and shape the root canal to accept a root canal filling material.

filling 1. The replacement material (gold or silver) used to restore that portion of a tooth that has decayed. *See also* core material (when referring to root canal therapy).

fixed appliance An appliance that is cemented by the dentist and thus cannot be removed by the patient.

flap surgery This technique involves reflecting (lifting) the gum away and then suturing (stitching) it back into place or into a new position that will be easier to clean.

fluoridation The addition of fluoride to water to strengthen teeth against tooth decay.

fluoridationist Those people in favor of the addition of fluoride to the public drinking water.

fluoride A chemical element that occurs naturally in great abundance in nature. When found or placed in correct amounts in drinking water, mouthwashes, toothpastes, etc., it helps prevent tooth decay.

fluoride disks Small disks attached to children's teeth that provide a continuous-feed fluoride supply for caries prevention.

fluorosis A discoloration of teeth from excessive fluoride in drinking water. This most frequently occurs when the water has natural fluoridation. It is characterized by lacy white lines (mottling).

focal infection theory An unproven theory of the 1910s that advocated oral bacteria could be trapped in a tooth during dental treatment, and then either the bacteria or the toxins they produce migrate to other parts of the body.

fracture A term used to describe a tooth that has been broken (either completely gone or just cracked).

FTC *See* Federal Trade Commission.

full denture An upper or lower denture used to replace all the teeth in a dental arch. It is supported by the dental ridge.

full-mouth survey A complete series of X-ray films (usually 18) taken to get a complete picture of all the existing teeth in the mouth.

functional appliance A dental appliance, usually used in orthodontics, that produces movement or stabilization of the teeth.

furcation Referring to the area between the tooth roots.

general anesthesia Sedation whereby a patient is not responsive to verbal commands. This is also termed unconscious sedation.

generalist Another term for a dentist who has not limited his practice to a dental specialty. Also called a general dentist.

general practitioner *See* generalist.

geriatric dentistry Dentistry for the elderly patient.

gingiva The technical term for the "gums."

gingivitis Inflammation of the gingival tissue. This is the beginning of periodontal disease.

glass ionomers A tooth-colored material made of fine glass powders that is used to restore teeth.

guided tissue regeneration (GTR) A process whereby a biocompatible material is used to isolate the defect from the tissue to allow the bone and connecting tissue to fill the space (bony defect).

gutta-percha A rubberlike material that is the most commonly used material today for filling root canals.

HA *See* hydroxylapatite.

handicapped patient Any patient who has either physical or psychological limitations.

health maintenance organization (HMO) An entity that contracts with subscribers and dependents to provide specified dental services for a defined period of time at a fixed per capita rate, regardless of the services provided.

hemisection A surgical endodontic procedure whereby root canal therapy is done on a multi-rooted tooth. Then, one or more roots and a portion of the crown are removed.

hepatitis B A disease transmitted by blood and blood products that is associated with liver disease.

herpes simplex These mouth sores are viral lesions that usually occur outside the mouth on the lips, but can be found in the roof of the mouth, the hard palate, and on the gum tissue. They are characterized by a feeling of fullness, burning, and itching before the vesicle develops.

HIV   An acronym for "human immunodeficiency virus."

HMO   *See* health maintenance organization.

human immunodeficiency virus (HIV)   A retrovirus transmitted by sexual contact, blood and blood products, or by an infected mother to her fetus or newborn at birth. This infection usually results in AIDS.

hydroxylapatite   A material used to increase the height and width of dental ridges. It is also used as a single-tooth root implant material. Sometimes known as "HA."

iatrogenesis   A tooth problem caused by a dental procedure. The problem may or may not be a result of negligence by the dentist.

immediate denture   A denture that is placed immediately after the teeth are extracted. The cost and care are usually more than for a "conventional" denture.

impacted   A tooth out of alignment from its normal path of eruption. Many impacted teeth never erupt.

implant   An extension of a tooth root or the replacement of a tooth by insertion of a metal post into the upper or lower dental ridges. This metal post serves to support the tooth crown.

implantology   An area of dentistry that involves tooth implants. It is *not* a specialty that is recognized by the ADA, so the training and experience varies.

impression   A replica of the mouth. Impressions are taken of teeth that have been prepared for a crown or dental ridges that need to be fitted for a denture so the lab can have an exact copy of the area. This enables the lab to make sure that they can make a crown or denture that fits exactly to the patient's existing tissue or tooth structure.

indemnity plan   An insurance company agrees to provide dental care for a specific population for an agreed period of time for an actuarially established per capita premium. The insurance company assumes the financial risk. Also known as a traditional or fee-for-service plan.

independent practice association (IPA)   An HMO model that involves contracting a group of independent dentists in private practice to provide a risk pool from which specific services are provided to eligible patients for a monthly capitation payment.

indirect pulp capping   The removal of as much decay as possible in a badly decayed tooth. A base is then placed over the excavated site. The idea is to prevent exposure of the dental pulp, which would make root canal therapy necessary. However, this procedure has a highly unpredictable long-term success rate.

individual practice association (IPA) An entity that is a form of HMO that contracts with providers to render services in their offices for a specific group of subscribers and dependents. The providers also treat patients not affiliated with the IPA. The providers assume the financial responsibility.

infective endocarditis (IE) A serious heart infection that can occur when microorganisms enter the bloodstream and make their way to the heart.

infiltration anesthesia Injection of a local anesthetic into the area to be treated. The numbing effect is not as extensive as in block anesthesia.

informed consent A statement for the patient to sign and date that explains in language understood by the patient all relevant information related to the proposed treatment. It should include alternatives and consequences of no treatment at all. This document is given to the patient to sign and date after the proposed treatement is discussed with the doctor who will do the procedure.

inlay A restoration that usually contains gold and alloys. This type of restoration restores the tooth without covering the cusps.

interceptive orthodontics Correction of minor oral conditions for the purposes of preventing or minimizing future orthodontic treatment.

internal derangement of the joint A term referring to a dislocated jaw, a displaced disc, or injury to the condyle.

intrapulpal injection A technique that involves placing the anesthetic directly into the pulp of the tooth.

intravenous (IV) sedation A method of managing extremely anxious patients through injecting sedatives (calming drugs) into the bloodstream. This should only be done by well-trained dentists who have the correct equipment, staff, etc.

intrusion A term used to describe a tooth that has been pushed up farther into the socket as a result of a blow

IPA *See* independent practice association.

IV sedation *See* intravenous sedation.

jaw relations The relationship of the upper jaw to the lower jaw when biting and chewing.

Keyes technique A nonsurgical system involving home care for the treatment of periodontal disease. This controversial technique has never been proven effective in controlled studies and is not recognized as useful by most periodontists.

laminated veneers A conservative technique involving the placement of a thin covering over discolored or broken teeth to improve their appearance. Laminated veneers are most frequently used on front teeth for cosmetic purposes.

242
▲

lasers   A light-generation source that emits concentrated energy that is collimated, allowing for the use of precision optics to transmit the generated energy. Each type of laser works on different wavelengths, which react differently on different tissues.

lateral head (X-ray) film   A large X-ray film usually taken by your orthodontist or oral surgeon to aid in planning treatment.

lead apron   A drape lined with lead that is put over the patient before an X ray is taken to protect the patient from being exposed to radiation. Many aprons also have lead collars that protect the thyroid gland from exposure to radiation.

lesion   The technical name of any sore. It could be either benign or malignant.

leukoplakia   A soft-tissue lesion that is characterized by a localized white patch or plaque. It is usually caused by irritation from a denture, broken tooth, or tobacco use.

lingual   The surface of a tooth in contact with the tongue; opposite to the buccal surface.

luxation   A term used to decribe a tooth injury in which the tooth has been displaced from its socket.

malformation   An abnormal anatomical structure.

malignant tumor   A cancerous growth.

malocclusion   A condition whereby the teeth are not correctly positioned, or when one or more of them is missing.

managed care plan   A dental insurance plan that controls expenditures of dental benefits by reducing the reimbursement levels, transferring the financial risk to the providers, limiting access to care, and restricting the type, level, and frequency of care.

managed fee-for-service plan   A dental insurance plan that pays the dentist directly for treatment on a fee-for-service basis. In return, the dentist agrees to certain contractural management provisions.

mandibular   A term referring to the lower jaw.

margin   The contact point between any restorative material and the tooth structure that abuts or lies under it. The margin of a properly placed restoration is smooth. There are no "catch points."

Maryland bridge   A type of tooth-replacing bridge that requires minimal reduction of adjacent teeth because it incorporatees wire mesh that attaches to each abutment tooth by a technique called bonding.

maxillary   A term referring to the upper jaw.

maxillofacial pain dysfunction syndrome (MPD)   Pain that often manifests itself as a toothache but is generally caused by spasms of the facial muscles.

maximum benefit   The insurance company sets a maximum amount they will pay each year in benefits for each person covered under the plan.

mesial   The surface of the tooth closest to the midline; opposite to the buccal surface.

midline   The imaginary vertical line that divides the face into two equal parts.

misplaced midline   An orthodontic condition whereby the midline of the upper and lower teeth do not match evenly.

mitral valve prolapse   A heart valve defect whereby patients with this problem should be premedicated with a regime of antibiotics as suggested by the American Heart Association before any dental treatment (including tooth cleaning) is started.

model   A likeness (replica) of a patient's teeth (made of plaster or stone) which can be use to construct tooth appliances or for studying the patient's occlusion (bite).

mouth guard   A plastic device (or sometimes made of a soft material) that fits over all the teeth in either the upper or lower arch and disbributes the forces of grinding equally.

MPD   An acronym for "maxillofacial pain dysfunction syndrome."

MVP   An acronym for "mitro valve prolapse."

myofascial pain   A regional, dull, muscular ache characterized by localized tender spots known as "trigger points" in the involved muscle and its associated area.

N-2   A paste root canal filling material banned from interstate shipping by the FDA. The active component is paraformaldehyde, which is caustic to the tissue.

National Institute of Dental Research (NIDR)   A national governmental health institute that studies and advises other governmental agencies in dental health policies. One of several dental research organizations.

National Institute of Health (NIH)   A national governmental health institute that studies and advises other governmental agencies on health-related policies.

Neo-cobefrin   A vasoconstrictor used in some anesthetics (e.g. 2% Carbocaine). Patients with heart disease should use Neo-cobefrin only on the advice of the patient's physician.

NIDR   *See* National Institute of Dental Research.

NIH   *See* National Institute of Health.

nitrous oxide/oxygen sedation   A method of managing anxious patients by allowing them to breathe the gas nitrous oxide through an inhalation mask to cause drowsiness, euphoria, amnesia, and slight analgesia.

nonvital tooth   A tooth that has had the pulp removed by root canal therapy.

obturate   The technical term used for filling a root canal.

occlude To close the two jaws so that the upper and lower teeth mesh (bite) together.

occlusal The chewing surface of a tooth.

occlusal adjustment Same as occlusal equilibration.

occlusal equilibration Adjustment of the biting relationships of the cusps of opposing teeth. Poor biting relationships may produce jaw or tooth pains.

occlusion The cuspal relationships of opposing arches of teeth. Also popularly called the "bite."

Occupational Health and Safety Administration (OSHA) A federal government agency concerned with the safety of employees in the workplace.

onlay A restoration usually containing gold and alloys that is used to restore (repair) a tooth by covering the cusps; hence, an onlay usually protects the tooth from fracture because a wedge effect is not created.

open bite A bite in which the teeth do not meet properly. This dental problem usually necessitates orthodontic treatment.

open panel This type of dental plan allows treatment to be provided to you and your dependents by any licensed dentist in your area. The benefits of the plan can either be paid to you or to the provider.

oral and maxillofacial surgery The dental specialty involving the diagnosis and treatment of diseases requiring surgical intervention.

oral candidiasis (thrush) A common localized infection of the inside of the mouth that is characterized by the formation of a smooth, creamy white or yellow plaque, but when wiped away the underlying mucosa tissue is red. It is associated with a decreased host defense caused by a variety of different drug therapies, systemic diseases, and local changes in the oral cavity.

oral pathology The dental specialty that is concerned with the diagnosis, causes, and treatment of oral diseases (e.g. oral cancer).

oral sedation A method of managing extremely anxious patients through oral administration of sedatives (calming drugs). This technique is usually considered safer than intravenous sedation.

oral surgery Now called oral and maxillofacial surgery.

orthodontic band A circular stainless-steel appliance cemented around the tooth. Brackets to hold orthodontic arch wires and elastics are attached to the band.

orthodontic bracket A square or rectangular shaped device that is attached to an orthodontic band to hold orthodontic wires and elastics.

orthodontics The dental specialty that is concerned with the diagnosis, causes, and treatment of improper occlusion ("crooked teeth"). Both adults and children may benefit from orthodontic treatment.

orthognathic surgery Surgery that involves changing the patient's facial bone structure. Also called cosmetic or reconstructive surgery.

OSHA An acronym for "Occupational Health and Safety Administration."

osseous (bone) surgery A technique that involves reshaping bone in the mouth.

osteointegration The bone integrates or bonds with the implant material.

osteomyelitis An infection around a tooth that extends into the bone supporting the roots of the tooth.

OTC *See* over-the-counter.

overbite A type of malocclusion involving a vertical or horizontal overlap. This problem usually requires orthodontic treatment.

overdenture A full denture that is secured to the roots of natural teeth that have had root canal therapy and crowns.

over-the-counter Any item(s) that are sold without a physician's or dentist's prescription. This term usually refers to a medicine.

panoramic radiograph An X ray (taken at three to five year intervals) to screen the lower portion of the face for "hidden" pathology not readily seen by other X-ray examinations.

paraformaldehyde The active chemical component of N-2, a paste root canal filling material. This chemical has been shown to cause severe bone and tissue destruction.

paresthesia Numbness of a portion of the face, usually the result of nerve damage from infection or other causes.

partial denture A removable tooth replacing prosthesis usually composed of a metal framework, clasps, and rests. It is both tooth and tissue supported. Partial dentures replace fewer teeth than a full denture and are used when a bridge is not suitable.

paste filling An injection system used to fill a root canal. The major difficulty of paste fillings is the inability of the dentist to confine the filling material to the root canal space.

pathology A disease. For example, a tissue that is infected. This disease can cause a localized and/or bodily infection.

pediatric dentist (also called a **pedodontist**) A dentist who is a specialist in dentistry for children.

peer review A review of a case by a special committee of volunteer dentists from the local dental society, usually at a patient's request. The purpose of the review is to resolve disputes between a dentist and a patient regarding the quality and/or appropriateness of the dental care provided.

perforation A "hole" or concavity in a vital tissue (tooth structure). If caused by nature, it is the result of an erosive process.

periapical   A term meaning that a problem originated from the apex (end) of the tooth root.

periapical film   An X-ray film that shows both the crown, root, and surrounding bone structure.

pericoronitis   Infection around a partially erupted tooth. Usually a pericoronitis is associated with a wisdom tooth.

peri-implantitis   This condition involves periodontal disease around implants.

periodontal disease   Pertaining to the gums and underlying bone.

periodontal ligament   The strong fibers that attach the tooth to supporting jaw bone.

periodontal ligament (PDL) injection   An infiltration technique for anesthetizing teeth. It is done by injecting anesthetic solution, under pressure, along the periodontal ligament between the tooth and its supporting bone.

periodontal pocket   A condition where the gum tissue recedes (pulls back) from the crown of the tooth, causing defects to form hold bacteria on the root surface of the tooth.

periodontal therapy   Treatment to correct periodontal disease.

periodontics   The specialty of dentistry that is concerned with the diagnosis, causes, prevention, and treatment of diseases of the gingiva (gums) and the supportive tissues of the teeth.

periodontitis   A dental term for advanced "gum disease."

periodontium   The supportive tissues of a tooth, including the gingiva and the underlying bone.

periradicular tissues   Those tissues surrounding the tooth roots.

phantom tooth pain (PTP)   A condition that involves chronic dental pain for no pathological reason. It usually occurs after endodontic treatment or in extraction sites.

PHS   *See* Public Health Service.

pin   A small metal post that is cemented into the crown portion of the tooth (never the canals) to aid in the retention of a filling material. The filling would not stay in the tooth without the pin(s).

pin-retained restoration   A restoration which has one or more pins placed into the dentin to retain the restorative material. Pins are placed when there is not enough tooth structure left to hold the filling.

pit-and-fissure sealant   *See* sealant.

plan maximum   A maximum allowance by a dental insurance plan for dental care in a fiscal/calendar year for each eligible person.

plaque   A colorless, sticky film composed of colonies of bacteria that constantly form and attach to the tooth.

pocket   *See* periodontal pocket.

pontic   A unit of a bridge that is the replacement for the missing teeth. Pontics are usually soldered to crowns that are placed on the abutment teeth.

porcelain   A material made of glass that is available in a variety of shades to make natural looking restorations for teeth.

post-and-core buildup   A small metal rod used to aid in lengthening a root canal–filled tooth and to provide support for the final crown. The post is placed within the upper two-thirds of the a root canal–treated tooth and a filling material is placed around it. This recreates the missing tooth structure so a metal or porcelain crown can be cemented in place.

posterior   A term used to refer to the back part of the mouth.

PPO   *See* preferred provider organization.

preauthorization   Essentially the same as predetermination.

predetermination   The amount an insurance company will allow for a procedure as determined prior to treatment.

preferred provider organization (PPO)   A group of dentists under contract to provide services at a discounted rate in exchange for access to that population. Also known as a contract dental organization (CDO).

pregnancy gingivitis   Gingival irritation in pregnant women. The cause is thought to be a result of female hormonal changes during pregnancy.

prophylaxis   A professional cleaning of the teeth that is completed by either a dentist or his hygienist in the dental office.

prosthodontics   The dental specialty dealing with both removable and fixed replacements for missing teeth.

protrusion   An orthodontic condition whereby the lower jaw and the upper teeth jut out.

provider   The dentist who is providing the dental treatment.

public health dentistry   A dental specialist whose work entails both being a dental service provider and, often, an adviser for matters of concern to the Public Health Service.

Public Health Service (PHS)   A public health provider and public health advisory body under the Department of Health and Human Services.

pulp   The soft, connective tissue inside the crown and roots of a tooth. The dental pulp is composed of cells, fibers, blood vessels, and nerves. It is this tissue that is removed during root canal therapy.

pulp capping   A technique that involves cleaning out the decay and placing a protective base over the exposed area. See direct and indirect pulp capping.

pulp chamber   The uppermost portion of the root canal system containing the bulk of pulp tissue. The pulp chamber occupies the space inside the tooth crown and is continuous with the space inside the tooth root.

pulpectomy   A procedure involving the removal of the entire dental pulp.

pulpotomy   A procedure involving the removal of the portion of the dental pulp in the crown of the tooth. A pulpotomy is sometimes done as an emergency procedure for relief of a toothache in an adult patient.

rebasing   A technique that involves making a new denture base that incorporates the existing denture tooth.

recurrent aphthous ulcers   Painful mouth sores that occur either singly or in clusters inside the mouth. They usually last 10 to 14 days. There is no consensus of opinion why these occur.

recurrent herpes labialis   *See* herpes simplex.

reline   A procedure involving the placement of a new, more closely fitting surface to an existing removable prosthetic appliance (e.g. denture). This should be done only by a dentist.

remineralize   A term meaning to harden.

removable appliance   An appliance (e.g. full or partial denture) for tooth replacement or tooth stabilization that can be taken in or out of the mouth.

replantation   A technique that involves replacing a tooth back into the socket after surgery has been performed on the tooth apex (end of root).

resins   Any number of tooth-colored filling materials including: bonded resins, microfill resins, or acid-etch resins.

resorption   The physiologic dissolving away of either tooth or bone structure.

restoration   Any filling that replaces tooth structure destroyed by dental caries.

rests   Metal components on partial dentures that keep the partial dentures from riding up and down. The indentations in the abutment teeth into which the rests fit are called "rest preparations."

retainer   A removable appliance to keep the teeth in proper position for a period of time after the braces are removed.

retraction   Pulling back (e.g. tissue).

retreatment   The primary root canal filling material is removed. The canals are cleaned, shaped, and then filled again.

retrofilling   A filling placed at the end of a root apex after the root has undergone an apicoectomy. The purpose of the filling is to seal the root apex.

ridge atrophy   Resorption or a decrease in the height of the dental ridge.

ridge augmentation   A surgical technique used to increase the ridge height and/or width.

root   The portion of the tooth below the crown and extending into the jawbone. The root is hollow and contains pulp tissue that is removed during root canal therapy.

root amputation   The removal of a tooth root. Root amputation differs from a hemisection in that root amputation does not entail removal of part of the crown.

root apex   The anatomical tip of the tooth root.

root canal   A term frequently used to mean root canal therapy. Also, more properly, the root canal is the space in the root occupied by pulp tissue.

root canal sealer   A paste used only to fill in the gaps between sections of the core material filling in a root canal.

root canal therapy   A procedure whereby the pulp of the tooth is removed and then, it is cleaned, shaped and, finally, filled. The term is frequently used synonymously with endodontic therapy.

root planing   A technique that involves the smoothing of the root surface so that plaque will not attach, thus enabling the gum tissue to reattach.

root resorption   The "eating away" or dissolving of areas both inside and outside the tooth root. This is particularly common after trauma.

rubber dam   A thin rubber sheet about six inches square that is stretched over a frame to isolate the tooth. This enables the tooth to be treated in a clean, dry environment.

scaling   A technique that involves the removal of plaque and calculus deposits from root surfaces below the gum line.

scheduled plans   Benefits are paid based on a percentage of a fee schedule that is set by the insurance company, also called usual and customary (UC).

Seal   *See* American Dental Association Seal of Acceptance.

sealant   An acid-etched resin that is placed primarily on the chewing surfaces of newly erupted permanent teeth to prevent caries on these surfaces.

self-insurance   A type of health insurance whereby an employer acts as the insuring agency. Benefits are paid directly to the employee after the dentist has rendered services.

silver cones   Small silver rods sometimes used as a core material to fill the root canal space. These are seldom used today. Also known as silver points.

silver points   *See* silver cones.

"space age" wires   Technologically advanced wires that are made of a super-elastic (nickel-titanium) material that exerts steady, gentle pressure on the teeth. This shortens treatment times and the amount of discomfort after adjustments.

spacing A gap between the teeth.

specialist A dentist with two or more years of training beyond dental school in an ADA-approved training program in one or more of the eight dental specialty areas.

splint 1. An appliance created to hold two or more teeth together to give added strength. Sometimes two crowns are soldered together to make a splint. 2. When used for dental-related pain (e.g. TMD or MFP), an appliance fabricated to cover all the teeth in either the upper or lower arch.

state dental society The same as a constituent dental society.

stress breaker A sophisticated device used in long-span bridges to reduce stresses. Stress breakers are used to reduce the chewing forces on poorly supported teeth, for example, periodontally diseased teeth that have lost much bone support.

subperiosteal An implant that consists of a metal frame that rests upon the jaw bone just below the gum tissue, instead of being placed directly into the jaw bone.

subscriber The person to whom the insurance company has issued a policy for insurance coverage. The immediate family members of the subscriber who are also eligible for insurance coverage under the subscriber's policy are know as dependents.

super-erupt A process whereby a tooth without an opposing tooth in the opposing arch continues to erupt. Age is not a factor in the process.

suture A stitch or the act of placing stitches after an operation.

table of allowances In dental insurance, the maximum dollar benefit for each specific dental procedure, regardless of the fee charged by the dentist.

tartar *See* calculus.

temporomandibular disorder (TMD) Any problem that prevents the complex system of structures in the TMJ from working together properly. It may result in cycles of pain, spasm (cramp), muscle tenderness, and damage to the tissue and joint.

temporomandibular joint (TMJ) The hinge joint that connects the upper and lower jaw bones. This enables you to chew.

temporomandibular splint *See* splint.

therapeutic A term describing any product that treats or prevents a disease.

thrush *See* oral candidiasis.

thyroid collar The top portion of a lead apron used during dental X-ray examination. The thyroid collar protects the thyroid gland.

titanium   The metal most frequently used in dental implants. The titanium in implants is generally the pure form of the metal.

TMJ   *See* temporomandibular joint.

topical anesthetic   An anesthetic applied by spraying or swabbing the surface tissue to provide some anesthetic to the surface tissue before it is injected to lessen the pain of the injection.

tort   A wrongful act resulting in the injury of individual(s) by other individual(s). Some form of damages are alleged and compensation is usually part of the settlement if the damages are determined to be valid. Dental malpractice cases are tort cases.

traditional plan   *See* indemnity plan.

tuberculosis (TB)   A highly contagious disease spread by airborne particles in the air. They are generated by people with TB who sneeze or cough.

UC   *See* usual and customary.

unconscious sedation   *See* general anesthesia.

undercutting   The method of mechanically securing a restoration (filling) that does not adhere to the walls of the cavity preparation. It involves creating convergent walls in the cavity space. Amalgam (silver) restorations are held in place by this technique.

unit   Each tooth and each pontic in a bridge.

universal precautions   Guidelines designed by the Center for Disease Control (CDC) and the Occupational Safety and Health Administration (OSHA) to protect all health professionals, staff, and patients from contracting all bloodborne pathogens. This includes HIV, hepatitis B, and AIDS.

unscheduled plan   The benefits are paid based on a percentile for the pervailing fees in a geographic area.

usual and customary rate (UCR)   The fee for a particular service that is determined by an insurance company to be usual and customary for your area of the country. Reimbursement for insurance claims is based on this rate. Also called a scheduled plan.

vasoconstrictor   Any chemical substance, such as epinephrine or Neocobefrin, which keeps the anesthetis in the area by diminishing the blood flow into or out of an area. An added advantage is it restricts bleeding during surgical procedures. Care should be taken before administering these chemicals (e.g. patients with severe heart disease).

vital tooth   A tooth that has a healthy pulp. It has not had root canal therapy.

xerostomia   A term for "dry mouth."

zinc oxide and eugenol   A powder (zinc oxide) and a liquid (eugenol) used as a base or temporary dental filling material.

Appendix A

UNITED STATES AND CANADIAN DENTAL SCHOOLS

United States

ALABAMA

University of Alabama
School of Dentistry
UAB Station
1919 7th Avenue South
Birmingham, Alabama 35294
(205) 934-4720

CALIFORNIA

University of the Pacific
School of Dentistry
2155 Webster Street
San Francisco, California 94115
(415) 929-6400

University of California,
  San Francisco
School of Dentistry
513 Parnassus Avenue
San Francisco, California 94143
(415) 476-1323

University of California, Los Angeles
School of Dentistry
Center for Health Sciences
Los Angeles, California 90024
(310) 825-7354

University of Southern California
School of Dentistry
University Park—MC 0641
Los Angeles, California 90089-0641
(213) 743-2800

Loma Linda University
School of Dentistry
Loma Linda, California 92350
(714) 796-0141

COLORADO

University of Colorado
School of Dentistry
4200 East Ninth Avenue, Box C-284
Denver, Colorado 80262
(303) 270-8773

CONNECTICUT

University of Connecticut
Center for Health Sciences
School of Dental Medicine
263 Farmington Avenue
Farmington, Connecticut 06032
(203) 679-2808

DISTRICT OF COLUMBIA

Howard University
College of Dentistry
600 W Street, N.W.
Washington, D.C. 20059
(202) 806-0440

FLORIDA

University of Florida
College of Dentistry
Box 405—JHMHC
Gainesville, Florida 32610
(904) 392-2946

Nova Southeastern University
College of Dental Medicine
3200 S. University Drive
Ft. Lauderdale, Florida 33328
(954) 723-1613

GEORGIA

Medical College of Georgia
School of Dentistry
1120 Fifteenth Street
Augusta, Georgia 30912
(404) 721-2117

ILLINOIS

Northwestern University
School of Dentistry
240 East Huron Street
Chicago, Illinois 60611
(312) 908-5932

Southern Illinois University
School of Dental Medicine
2800 College Avenue
Alton, Illinois 62002
(618) 474-7120

University of Illinois at Chicago
College of Dentistry
801 South Paulina Street
Chicago, Illinois 60612
(312) 996-1040

INDIANA

Indiana University
School of Dentistry
1121 West Michigan Street
Indianapolis, Indiana 46202
(317) 274-7957

IOWA

The University of Iowa
College of Dentistry
Dental Building
Iowa City, Iowa 52242
(319) 335-7144

KENTUCKY

University of Kentucky
College of Dentistry
800 Rose Street
Lexington, Kentucky 40536
(606) 233-5786

University of Louisville
School of Dentistry
Health Sciences Center
Louisville, Kentucky 40292
(502) 588-5293

LOUISIANA

Louisiana State University
School of Dentistry
1100 Florida Avenue
New Orleans, Louisiana 70119
(504) 947-9961

MARYLAND

University of Maryland
Baltimore College of Dental Surgery
School of Dentistry
666 West Baltimore Street
Baltimore, Maryland 21201
(410) 706-7462

MASSACHUSETTS

Harvard University
School of Dental Medicine

188 Longwood Avenue
Boston, Massachusetts 02115
(617) 432-1401

Boston University—Goldman
School of Graduate Dentistry
100 East Newton Street
Boston, Massachusetts 02118
(617) 638-4700

Tufts University
School of Dental Medicine
One Kneeland Street
Boston, Massachusetts 02111
(617) 956-5000

MICHIGAN

University of Detroit
School of Dentistry
2985 East Jefferson Avenue
Detroit, Michigan 48207
(313) 446-1800

University of Michigan
School of Dentistry
1234 Dental Building
Ann Arbor, Michigan 48109
(313) 763-6933

MINNESOTA

University of Minnesota
School of Dentistry
515 Delaware Street, S.E.
Minneapolis, Minnesota 55455
(612) 625-9982

MISSISSIPPI

The University of Mississippi
School of Dentistry
2500 North State Street
Jackson, Mississippi 39216
(601) 984-6000

MISSOURI

University of Missouri—Kansas City
School of Dentistry

650 East 25th Street
Kansas City, Missouri 64108
(816) 235-2100

NEBRASKA

Creighton University
Boyne School of Dental Science
2500 California Street
Omaha, Nebraska 68178
(402) 280-5060

University of Nebraska
College of Dentistry
Medical Center
40th & Holdrege Streets
Lincoln, Nebraska 68583
(402) 472-1344

NEW JERSEY

University of Medicine and
    Dentistry
New Jersey Dental School
100 Bergen Street
Newark, New Jersey 07103
(201) 456-4300

NEW YORK

Columbia University
School of Dental and Oral Surgery
630 West 168th Street
New York, New York 10032
(212) 305-2500

New York University
College of Dentistry
345 East 24th St.
New York, New York 10010
(212) 998-9800

State University of New York at
    Stony Brook
School of Dental Medicine
Health Sciences Center
Stony Brook, New York 11794
(516) 632-8950

State University of New York
at Buffalo
School of Dentistry
325 Squire Hall
Buffalo, New York 14214
(716) 831-2836

NORTH CAROLINA

University of North Carolina
School of Dentistry
104 Brauer Hall, CB#7450
Chapel Hill, North Carolina 27599
(919) 966-1161

OHIO

Ohio State University
College of Dentistry
305 West 12th Avenue
Columbus, Ohio 43210
(614) 292-9755

Case Western Reserve University
School of Dentistry
2123 Abington Road
Cleveland, Ohio 44106
(216) 368-3200

OKLAHOMA

University of Oklahoma
College of Dentistry
1001 N.E. Stanton L. Young
Oklahoma City, Oklahoma 73190
(405) 271-6326

OREGON

Oregon Health Sciences University
School of Dentistry
Sam Jackson Park
611 S.W. Campus Drive
Portland, Oregon 97201
(503) 494-8801

PENNSYLVANIA

Temple University
School of Dentistry

3223 N. Broad Street
Philadelphia, Pennsylvania 19140
(215) 221-2803

University of Pennsylvania
School of Dental Medicine
4001 West Spruce Street
Philadelphia, Pennsylvania 19104
(215) 898-8961

University of Pittsburgh
School of Dental Medicine
3501 Terrace Street
440 Salk Hall
Pittsburgh, Pennsylvania 15261
(412) 648-8900

PUERTO RICO

University of Puerto Rico
School of Dentistry
Medical Sciences Campus
G.P.O. Box 5067
San Juan, Puerto Rico 00936
(809) 758-2525

SOUTH CAROLINA

Medical University of South Carolina
School of Dentistry
171 Ashley Avenue
Charleston, South Carolina 29425
(803) 792-3811

TENNESSEE

Meharry Medical College
School of Dentistry
1005 18th Avenue North
Nashville, Tennessee 37208
(615) 327-6489

University of Tennessee
College of Dentistry
875 Union Avenue
Memphis, Tennessee 38163
(901) 528-6200

TEXAS

Baylor University
College of Dentistry
3302 Gaston Avenue
Dallas, Texas 75246
(214) 828-8100

The University of Texas
Health Sciences Center at Houston
Dental Branch
6516 John Freeman Avenue
Houston, Texas 77225
(713) 792-4021

The University of Texas
Health Science Center at
    San Antonio
School of Dentistry
7703 Floyd Curl Drive
San Antonio, Texas 78284
(512) 567-3160

VIRGINIA

Virginia Commonwealth University
School of Dentistry
Box 566—MCV Station

520 N. 12th St.
Richmond, Virginia 23298
(804) 786-9183

WASHINGTON

University of Washington
School of Dentistry
Health Sciences Mailstop SC-62
1959 N.E. Pacific
Seattle, Washington 98195
(206) 543-5982

WEST VIRGINIA

West Virginia University
School of Dentistry
The Medical Center North
Morgantown, West Virginia 26506
(304) 293-2521

WISCONSIN

Marquette University
School of Dentistry
604 North 16th Street
Milwaukee, Wisconsin 53233
(414) 288-7267

Canada

ALBERTA

University of Alberta
Faculty of Dentistry
3032 Dental-Pharmacy Center
Edmonton, Alberta T6G-2N8
(403) 432-3117

BRITISH COLUMBIA

University of British Columbia
Faculty of Dentistry
350-2194 Health Science Mall
Vancouver, British Columbia
    V6T-1W5
(604) 228-3562

MANITOBA

University of Manitoba
Faculty of Dentistry
780 Bannatyne Avenue
Winnipeg, Manitoba R3E-OW3
(204) 788-6631

NOVA SCOTIA

Dalhousie University
Faculty of Dentistry
5981 University Avenue
Halifax, Nova Scotia B3H-3J5
(902) 424-2275

ONTARIO

University of Toronto
Faculty of Dentistry
124 Edward Street
Toronto, Ontario M5G-1G6
(416) 979-4390

The University of Western Ontario
Faculty of Dentistry
London, Ontario N6A-5C1
(519) 661-3330

QUEBEC

Universite Laval
Ecole de Medecine Dentaire
Sainte Foy
Quebec, Quebec G1K-7P4
(418) 656-5303

McGill University
Faculty of Dentistry
3640 University Street
Montreal, Quebec H3A-2B2
(514) 398-7227

Universite de Montreal
Faculte de Medecine Dentaire
2900 Boulevard Edouard-Montpetit
C.P. 6209
Montreal, Quebec H3C-3J7
(514) 343-6005

SASKATCHEWAN

University of Saskatchewan
College of Dentistry
Saskatoon, Saskatchewan S7N-0W0
(306) 966-5056

Appendix B

National Dental Organization

American Dental Association
211 East Chicago Avenue
Chicago, Illinois 60611

The primary responsibility of the American Dental Association (ADA) is to assist your dentist. The first priority of the ADA staff is to handle telephone calls from dentists. Therefore, the ADA can honor only written requests from patients for patient information. Please *do not* call the ADA. Written requests from patients will be handled *promptly*.

Appendix C

State Dental Societies

ALABAMA

Alabama Dental Association
836 Washington Avenue
Montgomery, Alabama 36104
(205) 265-1684

ALASKA

Alaska Dental Society
3400 Spenard Road
Suite 10
Anchorage, Alaska 99503
(907) 277-4675

ARIZONA

Arizona State Dental Association
4131 N. 36th Street
Phoenix, Arizona 85018
(602) 957-4777

ARKANSAS

Arkansas State Dental Association
920 W. 2nd Street, Suite 103
Little Rock, Arkansas 72201
(501) 372-3368

CALIFORNIA

California Dental Association
1201 K Street

Sacramento, California 95853
(916) 443-3382

COLORADO

Colorado Dental Association
3690 S. Yosemite, Suite 100
Denver, Colorado 80237
(303) 740-6900

CONNECTICUT

Connecticut State Dental Association
62 Russ Street
Hartford, Connecticut 06106
(203) 278-5550

DELAWARE

Delaware State Dental Society
1925 Lovering Avenue
Wilmington, Delaware 19806
(302) 654-4335

DISTRICT OF COLUMBIA

District of Columbia Dental Society
502 C Street, N.E.
Washington, D.C. 20002
(202) 547-7613

FLORIDA

Florida Dental Association
1111 E. Tennessee Street
Suite 102
Tallahassee, Florida 32308
(904) 681-3629

GEORGIA

Georgia Dental Association
2801 Buford Hwy., Suite T-60
Atlanta, Georgia 30329
(404) 636-7553

HAWAII

Hawaii Dental Association
1000 Bishop Street
Suite 805
Honolulu, Hawaii 96813
(808) 536-2135

IDAHO

Idaho State Dental Association
1220 W. Hays Street
Boise, Idaho 83702
(208) 343-7543

ILLINOIS

Illinois State Dental Society
1010 Second Street
Springfield, Illinois 62701
(217) 525-1406

INDIANA

Indiana Dental Association
401 W. Michigan Street, Suite 1000
Indianapolis, Indiana 46202
(317) 634-2610

IOWA

Iowa Dental Association
505 Fifth Avenue, Suite 333
Des Moines, Iowa 50309
(515) 282-7250

KANSAS

Kansas Dental Association
5200 Huntoon Street
Topeka, Kansas 66604
(913) 272-7360

KENTUCKY

Kentucky Dental Association
1940 Princeton Drive
Louisville, Kentucky 40205
(502) 459-5373

LOUISIANA

Louisiana Dental Association
320 Third Street, Suite 201
Baton Rouge, Louisiana 70801
(504) 336-1692

MAINE

Maine Dental Association
Box 215
Manchester, Maine 04351
(207) 622-7900

MARYLAND

Maryland State Dental Association
6450 Dobbin Road
Columbia, Maryland 21045
(410) 964-2880

MASSACHUSETTS

Massachusetts Dental Society
83 Speen Street
Natick, Massachusetts 01760
(508) 651-7511

MICHIGAN

Michigan Dental Association
230 N. Washington Square, Suite 208
Lansing, Michigan 48933
(517) 372-9070

MINNESOTA

Minnesota Dental Association

2236 Marshall Avenue
St. Paul, Minnesota 55104
(612) 646-7454

MISSISSIPPI

Mississippi Dental Association
2630 Ridgewood Road
Jackson, Mississippi 39216
(601) 982-0442

MISSOURI

Missouri Dental Association
230 West McCarty Street
P.O. Box 1707
Jefferson City, Missouri 65102
(314) 634-3436

MONTANA

Montana Dental Association
P.O. Box 81
Helena, Montana 59624
(406) 443-2061

NEBRASKA

Nebraska Dental Association
3120 O Street
Lincoln, Nebraska 68510
(402) 476-1704

NEVADA

Nevada Dental Association
6889 West Charleston Blvd., Suite B
Las Vegas, Nevada 89117
(702) 255-4211

NEW HAMPSHIRE

New Hampshire Dental Society
Box 2229
Concord, New Hampshire 03301
(603) 225-5961

NEW JERSEY

New Jersey Dental Association
One Dental Plaza

North Brunswick, New Jersey 08902
(908) 821-9400

NEW MEXICO

New Mexico Dental Association
3736 Eubank Blvd. N.E., Suite 1A
Albuquerque, New Mexico 87111
(505) 294-1368

NEW YORK

Dental Society of the State of New York
7 Elk Street
Albany, New York 12207
(518) 465-0044

NORTH CAROLINA

North Carolina Dental Society
P.O. Box 12047
Raleigh, North Carolina 27605
(919) 832-1222

NORTH DAKOTA

North Dakota Dental Association
Box 1332
Bismarck, North Dakota 58502
(701) 223-8870

OHIO

Ohio Dental Association
1370 Dublin Road
Columbus, Ohio 43215
(614) 486-2700

OKLAHOMA

Oklahoma Dental Association
629 W. Interstate 44, Service Road
Oklahoma City, Oklahoma 73118
(405) 848-8873

OREGON

Oregon Dental Association
17898 S.W. McEwan Road
Portland, Oregon 97224
(503) 620-3230

PENNSYLVANIA

Pennsylvania Dental Association
3501 North Front Street
Box 3341
Harrisburg, Pennsylvania 17110
(717) 234-5941

PUERTO RICO

Puerto Rico Dental Association
Domenech Avenue, Suite 200
Hato Rey, Puerto Rico 00918
(809) 764-1969

RHODE ISLAND

Rhode Island Dental Association
200 Centerville Place
Warwick, Rhode Island 02886
(401) 732-6833

SOUTH CAROLINA

South Carolina Dental Association
120 Stonemark Lane
Columbia, South Carolina 29210
(803) 750-2277

SOUTH DAKOTA

South Dakota Dental Association
Box 1194
Pierre, South Dakota 57501
(605) 224-9133

TENNESSEE

Tennessee Dental Association
Box 120188
Nashville, Tennessee 37212
(615) 383-8962

TEXAS

Texas Dental Association
Box 3358
Austin, Texas 78764
(512) 443-3675

UTAH

Utah Dental Association
1151 East 3900 South
Suite B-160
Salt Lake City, Utah 84124
(801) 261-5315

VERMONT

Vermont State Dental Society
132 Church Street
Burlington, Vermont 05401
(802) 864-0115

VIRGIN ISLANDS

Virgin Islands Dental Association
Box 10422
St. Thomas, Virgin Islands 00801
(809) 775-9110

VIRGINIA

Virginia Dental Association
Box 6906
Richmond, Virginia 23230
(804) 358-4927

WASHINGTON

Washington State Dental Association
2033 Sixth Avenue, Suite 333
Seattle, Washington 98121
(206) 448-1914

WEST VIRGINIA

West Virginia Dental Association
300 Capitol Street, Suite 1002
Charleston, West Virginia 25301
(304) 344-5246

WISCONSIN

Wisconsin Dental Association
111 E. Wisconsin Avenue,
Suite 1300
Milwaukee, Wisconsin 53202
(414) 276-4520

WYOMING

Wyoming Dental Association
330 South Center Street,
Suite 322
Casper, Wyoming 82601
(307) 234-0777

Canadian Dental Associations

Alberta Dental Association
101-8230 105 Street
Edmonton, Alberta
T6E 5H9
(403) 432-1012

College of Dental Surgeons of
British Columbia
500-1765 West 8th Avenue
Vancouver, British Columbia
V6J 1J9
(604) 736-3621

Manitoba Dental Association
103-698 Corydon Avenue
Winnipeg, Manitoba
R3M OX9
(204) 453-0055

New Brunswick Dental Society
Suite 11, 403 Regent Street
Fredericton, New Brunswick
E3B 3X6
(506) 452-8575

Newfoundland Dental Association
211 LeMarchant Road
St. John's, Newfoundland
A1C 2H5
(709) 579-2362

Nova Scotia Dental Association
604-5991 Spring Garden Road
Halifax, Nova Scotia
B3H 1Y6
(902) 420-0088

Ontario Dental Association
4 New Street
Toronto, Ontario
M5R 1P6
(416) 922-3900

Dental Association of P.E.I.
184 Belvedere Avenue
Charlottetown, Prince Edward Island
CIA 2ZI
(902) 894-4022

Association des Chirurgiens
Dentistes du Quebec
1425-425 Ouest Boul. de
Maisonneuve
Montreal (Quebec)
H3A 3G5
(514) 282-1425

College of Dental Surgeons of
Saskatchewan
101-500 Spadina Cres. E.
Saskatoon, Saskatchewan
S7K 4H9
(306) 244-5072

Index

Italicized letters *f* and *t* following page numbers
indicate figures and tables, respectively.